W9-DEC-702

The Fifteen Minute Hour:
Therapeutic Talk in Primary Care

The Fifteen Minute Hour: Therapeutic Talk in Primary Care

MARIAN R. STUART PhD

Professor Emeritus of Family Medicine
University of Medicine and Dentistry of New Jersey
Robert Wood Johnson Medical School

and

JOSEPH A. LIEBERMAN III MD, MPH

Professor of Family Medicine
Jefferson Medical College of Thomas Jefferson University, Philadelphia, PA

Foreword by

ROBERT E. RAKEL MD

Professor, Department of Family and Community Medicine
Baylor College of Medicine, Houston, TX

Radcliffe Publishing
Oxford • New York

Radcliffe Publishing Ltd
18 Marcham Road
Abingdon
Oxon OX14 1AA
United Kingdom

www.radcliffe-oxford.com
Electronic catalogue and worldwide online ordering facility.

British Library Cataloguing in Publication Data

A catalogue record for this book is available from the British Library.

ISBN-13: 978 184619 288 3

Typeset by Pindar New Zealand, Auckland, New Zealand
Printed and bound by Cadmus Communications, USA

Contents

Foreword

The fact that this book has progressed to a fourth edition confirms the usefulness of these techniques to those of us in primary care. Although the basic concepts presented are similar to earlier editions, much new material has been added to make these principles and techniques more useful to the primary care health professional.

Today, perhaps more than ever before, stress plays a role in everyone's life. It affects daily activities, influences the way symptoms are perceived, and detracts from quality of life. It is a component of every illness and must be addressed no matter what the presenting symptoms or how "organic" the illness may be. In fact, the person with a specific organic illness may need more help addressing the emotions related to that illness than someone with a purely "functional" disease. Our responsibility as primary care professionals is to help our patients manage this stress and recognize when it calls for specific therapeutic measures.

The reader will notice the frequent reference to caring and compassion, which are essential to providing good primary care. Caring implies empathy, which is the ability to participate in the feelings of another. Compassion is the wish for the other to be free of their suffering and is associated with a sense of commitment, responsibility, and respect. Of the three attributes of prevention, curing, and caring, caring is the most important.

An insightful medical student said, "I hope that someday my words will be as healing as my technical knowledge." Too often our caring is supplanted by managing, and the art of listening is taken over by technological procedures. Listening is essential to caring, but it is not passive. Bernard Lown, in *The Lost Art of Healing*[1] says that "One must be an active listener to hear an unspoken problem." Effective communication depends much more on our ability to be a good listener than on what we say to the patient. Truly listening is a form of respect and is essential to developing trust.

A primary care practitioner who is locked into the biologic model is much less effective than one who appropriately incorporates the psychological and social aspects of health care. The mind-body approach to medicine is not a dichotomy but a dualism that promotes improved patient care and views the relationship with the patient as a complex interaction involving emotional, relational, and belief systems. We can treat a malfunctioning organ system but true healing occurs when we give relief to a distressed human being.

The biopsychosocial approach presented here, although an accurate term, may be a turn-off because of its complexity. However, it is the essence of looking at the whole patient and recognizing the myriad of factors that can affect one's mental and physical well being. Our preoccupation with biomedical medicine has not only diminished the attention given to the biopsychosocial but, as some believe, it may have denigrated it as irrelevant.

The BATHE technique described in Chapter 4 allows the professional to incorporate the principal features of psychosocial medicine into the patient interview and achieve a better outcome than those who are stuck in the disease-oriented mode.

Patients seen in primary care often present with vague, undifferentiated symptoms. The identification of potentially serious problems in their early, undifferentiated stage is one of the most difficult and challenging tasks in medicine.

This book is a valuable resource for primary care physicians and all health professionals involved in providing primary care to patients. It contains many simple and practical techniques that are useful in practice.

Robert E. Rakel MD
Professor
Department of Family and Community Medicine
Baylor College of Medicine
Houston, TX
July 2008

Reference

1. Lown B. *The Lost Art of Healing: practicing compassion in medicine.* New York: Ballantine Books; 1999.

Preface

The publication of this fourth edition of *The Fifteen Minute Hour* by Radcliffe Publishing is a source of great satisfaction to us. Our purpose in writing this book, which has not changed since our first edition in 1986, is to convince you that by routinely incorporating therapeutic talk into your practice, you can solve and often prevent many problems. During the years since publication of the first edition, many things have changed. In earlier editions we speculated about a number of mind-body connections that have since been substantiated by research. The increase in terrorism around the world has compromised people's basic sense of safety. Evidence-based medicine, electronic communications, the plethora of information on the internet, cost control, cultural diversity, and other societal trends have affected the delivery of medical care. In spite of all these changes, the importance of the practitioner-patient relationship remains a constant. The approaches described in this text are designed not only to enhance the therapeutic relationship, but also to make your practice more productive and pleasurable.

The book has grown out of our combined 70+ years of clinical practice and experience in teaching doctors training in the specialty of Family Medicine, practicing physicians, nurse practitioners, and other primary care providers in the art of therapeutic talk. In the 22 years since the publication of the first edition of *The Fifteen Minute Hour*, we have heard from many enthusiastic practitioners in the United States, Australia, Brazil, Canada, Denmark, Israel, Malta, the United Kingdom, and elsewhere who have assimilated our techniques into their practices. We were delighted when the second edition was translated into Japanese, and the third edition was translated into Korean, because this attested to the multicultural relevance of our techniques. The overwhelming consensus is that the strategies work: patients respond, practitioners save time, provider-patient relationships become richer, and everyone feels a little less stressed out.

Although our techniques will certainly increase your ability to recognize and treat emotional problems, this is not a psychiatry text. It is also not a text on providing in-depth psychotherapy or long-term counseling although it will enhance your ability to recognize and manage common emotional conditions resulting from the stress of living in the 21st century. You will be able to address patients' concerns often at an early and manageable state. Incorporating useful knowledge from psychology and psychotherapy into your medical practice will help you become more effective in dealing with the emotional component of problems patients bring to the primary care practitioner and leave you feeling more satisfied.

When *The Fifteen Minute Hour* was first published, addressing psychological issues related to the patient's health status was not seen as critical. Max Planck has been quoted as explaining that "a new scientific truth does not triumph by convincing its opponents and making them see the light, but rather because its opponents eventually die, and a new generation grows up that is familiar with it." We have been preaching this "gospel" for over 22 years. You are our new generation. We hope that you will master our simple techniques to deal effectively with the psychological dimensions of patient care. If you already focus on patients' psychosocial problems or would like to do so more efficiently, this book will provide you with background material to help you apply universal principles. We will point out what actually works in practice to improve patients' functioning. Furthermore, we will provide specific suggestions, approaches to therapeutic interventions, and particular phrases that we have developed, practiced, taught, and tested for over 30 years. We now have evidence to document that our techniques increase patient satisfaction[1,2] and improve practitioner-patient relationships[3] without adding significantly to the length of the visit.[4]

Our way is not necessarily the only true, good, or beautiful way to make therapeutic interventions, but it is a pragmatic and flexible approach that is easily learned, and it works! Also, it is designed to fit into a regular office visit of 15 minutes or less without requiring lengthy therapy sessions.

We strongly recommend that you read this book from beginning to end. Early chapters provide the theoretical background and rationale, and subsequent chapters focus on putting this knowledge into action. In essence, this is a how-to book. We aim to help you develop skills that will benefit both you and your patient. We provide some effective tools for use in your practice, and we explain exactly how to use them. These tools require less investment of time and energy than you might imagine.

There are many schools of therapy. We are not preaching a dogma, nor do we have the need to establish a true religion in this area. We are quite comfortable with practical eclecticism because it works, and primary care practitioners desperately need techniques that work. We invite you to apply our techniques and empirically confirm their usefulness for yourself. In essence, we are saying, "Try it, you'll like it."

John Godfrey Saxe, a Vermont lawyer and humorist, wrote "The Blind Men and the Elephant"[5] over 100 years ago. This poem was based on an Indian tale thought to date back thousands of years. It still seems most applicable.

It was six men of Indostan
   To learning much inclined,
Who went to see the Elephant
   (Though all of them were blind)
That each by observation
   Might satisfy his mind.

The First approached the Elephant,
   And happening to fall
Against his broad and sturdy side,
   At once began to bawl:
"God bless me! but the Elephant
   Is very like a wall!"

The Second, feeling of the tusk,
   Cried, "Ho! what have we here
So very round and smooth and sharp?
   To me 'tis mighty clear
This wonder of an Elephant
   Is very like a spear!"

The Third approached the animal,
   And happening to take
The squirming trunk within his hands,
   Thus boldly up and spake:
"I see," quoth he, "the Elephant
   Is very like a snake!"

The Fourth reached out an eager hand,
   And felt about the knee
"What most this wondrous beast is like
   Is mighty plain," quoth he;
"'Tis clear enough the Elephant
   Is very like a tree!"

The Fifth who chanced to touch the ear,
   Said: "E'en the blindest man
Can tell what this resembles most;
   Deny the fact who can,
This marvel of an Elephant
   Is very like a fan!"

The Sixth no sooner had begun
   About the beast to grope

Than, seizing on the swinging tail
    That fell within his cope,
"I see," quoth he, "the Elephant
    Is very like a rope!"

And so these men of Indostan
    Disputed loud and long,
Each in his own opinion
    Exceeding stiff and strong,
Though each was partly in the right,
    And all were in the wrong!

Different schools of psychology and psychiatry view the patient and the patient's problems from different perspectives. Each provides a small piece of useful insight. Collectively these fragments form a tool kit which can be used to reduce patients' suffering, prevent many physical and psychological illnesses, and help patients structure more satisfying lives for themselves and their loved ones.

In writing this book, we have tried to present a coherent whole. Each chapter builds on the previous one, and illustrative clinical examples appear throughout the text. The case material, including all new examples, is based entirely on actual encounters, although we have changed names and altered some details to guarantee patients' confidentiality. In revising the text for this edition, we have considered the many thoughtful critiques and reviews of *The Fifteen Minute Hour* and have clarified and expanded important sections and eliminated extraneous material.

Chapter 1 presents important background material. We discuss how the current understanding of the body-mind connection supports the need to address a medical patient's psychological issues, why the primary care practitioner is qualified to enter this realm, and how our therapeutic interventions differ from those of a traditional psychiatrist. Chapter 2 details patients' reactions to stress and provides a theoretical basis for the effectiveness of the type of interventions we are promoting. We bring together research findings from a variety of sources, some of which may be new to you, and try to establish a strong foundation.

Chapter 3 focuses on Cognitive Behavioral Therapy (CBT) and other modalities that lend themselves for use in a brief office visit. We discuss the elements common to all schools of psychotherapy and bring in several new concepts to simplify the process of inducing positive change. Chapter 4 introduces the BATHE technique as a basic structure to obtain psychosocial data, support patients and build a therapeutic relationship. Chapters 5, 6 and 7 provide a rich variety of techniques that can be used in brief, follow-up counseling sessions with patients. We have expanded material dealing with hypochondriasis, anxiety, depression, grief, potential suicide, and issues related to children and teens.

Chapter 8, newly created for this fourth edition, presents material from the field of Positive Psychology and shows how to potentially enhance patients' health by focusing them on the affirmative aspects of their lives and relationships. It is our hope that the modified techniques and applications we outline will enrich the experience of both practitioners and patients. Chapter 9 suggests ways that incorporating our material will improve the office environment, increase patient satisfaction, and prevent staff and practitioner burnout. Throughout the book, we have added evidence-based material related to behavioral medicine. Chapter 10 projects our vision of what is possible for primary care practice given widespread acceptance and application of these ideas.

We hope you will enjoy reading *The Fifteen Minute Hour*. Please have fun with it. Your patients will thank you many times over.

Marian R. Stuart PhD
Joseph A. Lieberman III MD, MPH
July 2008

References

1. Jones K, Major G, Marvel K. Counseling patients for lifestyle change: a comparison of two methods. *Proceedings of the Society of Teachers of Family Medicine*, Seattle, WA. May 1998.
2. Leiblum SL, Schnall E, Seehuus M, *et al.* To BATHE or not to BATHE: patient satisfaction with visits to their family medicine physician. *Fam Med.* 2008; **40**(6): 407-11.
3. Kallerup H. Patient's and doctors' considerations about using communication strategies. *Proceedings of the 24th Annual Meeting of the North American Primary Care Research Group*; 1996 Nov 3–6; Vancouver, BC.
4. Searight HR. Efficient counseling techniques for the primary care physician. *Prim Care Clin Office Pract.* 2007; **34**: 551–70.
5. Saxe JG. *Clever Stories of Many Nations: rendered in rhyme.* Boston: Ticknor & Fields; 1865.

About the Authors

Marian R. Stuart PhD is Professor Emeritus of Family Medicine at the University of Medicine and Dentistry of New Jersey-Robert Wood Johnson Medical School. After 30 years of teaching medical students, doctors in graduate medical training, faculty and practicing physicians, she has limited her activities to consulting, faculty development and private practice as a Licensed Psychologist in Morristown, NJ. She is in great demand as a speaker on communications skills, stress management, successful aging, forgiveness, and medical education. She has lectured and given workshops in most areas of the United States as well as in the UK, Canada, Denmark and Israel. Dr. Stuart is the recipient of the 1997 Society of Teachers of Family Medicine Excellence in Education Award, and a charter member of the Stuart D Cook MD Master Educators Guild of UMDNJ. In 2002 the American Academy of Family Physicians made her an Honorary Member, an extraordinary achievement for a psychologist.

Dr. Stuart has three grown children and four grandchildren. In her leisure time she is an avid environmentalist and enjoys a variety of outdoor activities and dance with her life partner, Keith.

Joseph A. Lieberman III MD, MPH is Professor of Family Medicine at Jefferson Medical College, of Thomas Jefferson University, in Philadelphia, Pennsylvania. He received his BS degree from Georgetown University, his MD from Jefferson Medical College and his Masters of Public Health from UMDNJ/Rutgers University. He completed his Internship at Sacred Heart Hospital and his Fellowship at the Institute of Medicine of the National Academy of Sciences in Washington, DC.

Prior to accepting his present position, at his Alma Mater, he was Professor and Chairman of the Department of Family Medicine at UMDNJ-Robert Wood Johnson Medical School. Prior to that he had been in the private practice of Family Medicine for 10 years, which had immediately followed his service in the Medical Corps of the United States Air Force.

A frequent contributor to the medical literature, his publications and presentations of books, book chapters, papers, educational CDs, audio and video tapes, and films number into the hundreds. He also serves on the editorial boards and editorial review boards of a number of prestigious medical journals including, but not limited to, *JAMA, The Journal of Clinical Psychiatry, The Journal of Family Practice* and *The Journal of the American Board of Family Medicine.*

Dr. Lieberman has also served as President of both the New Jersey and Delaware Academies of Family Physicians and he has twice received both the Exceptional Merit Award from UMDNJ and the Medical Society of Delaware's President's Award as well as a special Tribute from the State of Delaware's Senate and House of Representatives.

Acknowledgments

The authors wish to recognize and express appreciation to the many people who made meaningful contributions to this book and its earlier editions. We would first like to thank the following physicians: Maria Auletta MD, Bryant Nguyen MD, Hana Chaim DO, Alicia Dermer MD, Steven Frank DO, Joan Gopin MD, Patricia Janku MD, Naomi Kolb MD, Ronald Lau MD, Yves Morency MD, Jay D. Patel MD, Jean Plover MD, Jamie L. Reedy MD, MPH, Andrew Sachere MD, Yasser Soliman MD, Roger Thompson MD, Harvey Weingarten MD and Tanya Zaremba MD for practicing our methods and contributing experiential clinical material. We would also like to acknowledge our colleagues: Beatrix Hamm MD, PhD, Robert C. Like MD, David E. Swee MD, and Alfred F. Tallia for their continuing support and encouragement. Special thanks to Afton L. Hassett PsyD, Margaret Chan PhD and Anu Kotay PhD for their research and editorial assistance. We would also like to thank Ms. Robin Covington and Dr. Vikram Gupta without whose skill and support our work could not have been completed. Finally, we would like to thank our editor, Ms. Gillian Nineham, for her clear vision, her expert guidance and her support.

CHAPTER 1

The Body-Mind and the Role of the Primary Care Practitioner

A recent study determined that worrying about terrorism takes a toll on peoples' hearts. People who were most fearful about the possibility of attacks as related to national alerts were three to five times more likely to develop a new cardiovascular ailment.[1]

Studies are proliferating that clearly establish the connection between peoples' health, their emotional states, and the circumstances of their lives. Since emotional problems often manifest as physical problems and physical problems usually have emotional consequences, physical and emotional problems must be addressed in an integrated manner. Whether or not the practitioner invites or even desires it, patients often expect help with emotional problems along with physical problems. The practitioner becomes a therapist by default. In this chapter we will discuss the connection between mental and physical health as it is currently understood, the qualifications of primary care practitioners to address patients' emotional issues, and how this type of intervention differs from treatment by a mental health specialist.

A considerable body of literature documents primary care as the de facto mental health care system in the United States and the pervasive nature of mental health care needs in the community.[2,3] In many communities the primary care practitioner is the only professional, with training in mental health, available to patients.[4,5] However, even in the absence of psychiatric conditions per se, our emphasis is on promoting health by mitigating the effects of psychological stress on the physical condition of the patient.

One of the beauties of primary care practice is the diversity of patient problems. This also gives rise to profound challenges, particularly regarding the behavioral, and in more extreme cases, the psychiatric aspects of this type of practice. Effective health care mandates enabling clinicians to provide appropriate psychiatric interventions in order to diminish the suffering of their patients. One of the more effective ways to do this is to address the sources of

1

patients' distress and not just the effects. As George Engel pointed out over a quarter century ago:

> The crippling flaw of the (traditional medical) model is that it does not include the patient and his attributes as a person, as a human being. The biomedical model can make provision neither for the person as a whole nor for data of a psychological or social nature, for the reductionism and mind-body dualism on which the model is predicated requires that these must first be reduced to physicochemical terms before they can have meaning. Hence, the very essence of medical practice perforce remains "art" and beyond the reach of science.[6]

THE TENSION BETWEEN THE SCIENTIFIC METHOD AND PATIENTS' NEEDS

Patients generally arrive at the primary care office knowing only that they do not feel well and have symptoms. After a series of maneuvers and studies, patients are informed of a purported cause for their symptoms. If this is amenable to a specific therapy, they will have their symptoms relieved and be considered cured. The practitioner is gratified that the treatment is successful and the patient is satisfied and grateful since the particular problem has been ameliorated. More commonly, however, the patient's symptoms are part of a larger entity. Patients are complex, multidimensional human beings, and they bring a variety of problems to the clinician; some are quite obvious, while others take the form of hidden agendas.[7] If the practitioner simply focuses on the biomedical aspects that are presented, this one-dimensional view may prevent an accurate diagnosis of the patient's real problems.

The presenting problem (which can usually be handled with little difficulty) may not be the main reason for the patient's visit. A substantial body of literature documents that people do not visit clinicians simply for relief of organic disorders but also go to the primary care providers because of life stress, psychiatric disorders, social isolation and informational needs.[8] Too often patients are only treated with pills that relieve their most obvious symptoms but do not treat the underlying condition. By "turning off" the symptom (which is a signal that something is wrong) the clinician removes the evidence without addressing the problem. By analogy, if we were to turn off the bell on our telephone, we would never know when someone was calling and therefore we could not respond by either giving or receiving information.

INTERRELATIONSHIP BETWEEN PHYSICAL AND PSYCHOLOGICAL HEALTH

Recent research clearly substantiates the inadequacy of the reductionistic method and the traditional biological approach in the evaluation of symptoms. The psyche and the soma are so closely related that imbalances in either one can produce symptoms or disease in the other.[9–11] These investigations indicate conclusively that the soma does not function in a vacuum, but rather, that the psyche and the soma are so closely related that imbalances in either one can produce symptoms or disease in the other. Indeed, there has been a geometric progression in the production of studies of stress related disorders. A recent article in *The Journal of the American Medical Association* documents a significant increase in expenditures related to treatment of back and neck pain between 1997 and 2005 and attests to the limits of physicians' ability to successfully improve patients' health status.[12] An earlier study compared a biopsychosocial approach to conventional biomedical treatment of patients with low back pain finding that although both groups demonstrated similar improvement at three months, the biopsychosocial group had significantly better results at six months. Furthermore, by the end of two years, 59% of the biopsychosocial group required no sick leave due to low back pain compared to 10% in the biomedical group.[13]

Patients' psychological responses to diagnosis or treatment can have a significant impact on the course of their disease. An early study by Greer, Morris, and Pettingale found that women diagnosed as having breast cancer who expressed anger and hostility had a better prognosis than those who passively and helplessly accept their disease.[14] D. Spiegel and his colleagues were absolutely amazed to find that women with breast cancer who were in support groups not only had a much better quality of life (as had been expected), but survived significantly longer than women in the control group.[15] Since these initial studies, much similar research has been conducted leading reviewers to conclude that emotional processes can affect cancer progression, quality of life, and survival.[16,17]

Effects of Stress on the Immune System

R.W. Bartrop and his colleagues were the first to report on the mechanisms involved in the well-known mortality risk following bereavement.[18] A prospective study published in *The Journal of the American Medical Association* replicated their study by monitoring the immune system of husbands of women with breast cancer, and found a highly significant suppression of lymphocyte function to specific antigens within one month of the spouse's death. This suppression lasted for a period of 14 months after bereavement and was not due to pre-existing conditions.[19] Kiecolt-Glaser and her colleagues observed a consistent finding across multiple labs that negative emotions are related to (1) poorer response to vaccines, (2) increased susceptibility to illness, and (3) longer lasting infections.[20]

Over the last 20 years, the field of psychoneuroimmunology (PNI) has provided insight into the mechanisms involved in the relationship between psychological factors and the pathogenesis of disease. The most compelling evidence for the bi-directional communication between the nervous and immune systems has been the findings that:

1. nerve endings can be found in the tissues of the immune system
2. central nervous system (CNS) changes alter immune response and an immune response alters CNS activity
3. an immune response alters hormone and neurotransmitter levels and vice versa
4. lymphocytes are able to produce neurotransmitters and hormones
5. psychological factors may render one vulnerable to the progression of autoimmune disease, infectious disease, and cancer
6. immunologic reactivity can be influenced by stress, hypnosis, and classical conditioning.[21,22]

Other Body-mind Interactions

Patients who have a tendency to interpret illness in a pessimistic fashion and to respond to symptoms in an all-or-nothing manner are more prone to develop irritable bowel syndrome (IBS) after a bout of gastroenteritis especially when they are experiencing high levels of stress and anxiety.[23] Researchers have observed that when patients with diabetes are exposed to a stressor, they experience a delay in glucose metabolism after eating.[24] The emotional and physical gut connection can also be clearly demonstrated even in healthy patients.[25]

The pathophysiological links between behavioral factors and cardiovascular disease and other life threatening illnesses are increasingly being studied.[26] For example, depression has been shown to be a risk factor for cardiac disease.[27] Studies focusing on the role of psychosocial influences on morbidity and mortality and myocardial infarction are proliferating.[28,29] Recent literature supports a strong relationship between negative emotions, life stress, and inadequate social support and coronary heart disease.[30–32] Although these findings support the notion of a causal relationship, conclusive proof is still pending. Instead, psychological factors should be considered important (modifiable) risk factors. And if the psyche and the soma were not integrally related, none of these effects would occur.

Mental Health and the Traditional Medical Model

It is an unfortunate fact that the fractured American health care system does not provide adequately for mental health care. However, even in countries that provide comprehensive and universal health care, it is critically important for clinicians to develop skills to identify specific problems, address patients' needs in a time-effective manner, provide initial support and then refer patients for further treatment, when necessary.

In this book, we present strategies to help primary care practitioners provide effective psychosocial treatment in the context of a standard office practice. These strategies, coupled with good medical practice, should enable the practitioner to treat patients, not diagnoses and help people make and maintain lifestyle changes to promote their physical and mental health.

The traditional paradigm of medical treatment is built around the following concepts:

1. patients suffer from diseases that can be categorized
2. diseases are independent of the persons suffering from them
3. each disease has a specific causal agent
4. the physician's task is to diagnose and prescribe
5. the correct disease can be determined through a process of differential diagnosis
6. the patient is a passive recipient of this process and
7. mental and physical diseases can be considered separately, except in specific psychosomatic diseases where the mind appears to act on the body.[33]

Limitations of the Traditional Medical Model

The three most glaring limitations of this model are the illness/disease anomaly, the specific etiology anomaly and the mind/body anomaly. The first concerns the incidence of illness without disease. Studies of abdominal pain have shown that specific diagnoses were obtained in less than 50% of cases. Headache, chest pain, back pain, and other illness often present in the absence of clear-cut, identifiable disease.[34]

The second anomaly concerns the general susceptibility to disease that is evidenced by some individuals. Why is it that 25% of the patients have 75% of the illness? If diseases truly had specific etiologies, then it would seem likely that every person would have an even chance of contracting them. However, this is not the case. In subsequent chapters, we will be discussing some of the factors that make people either more or less vulnerable.

The third anomaly concerns the effects of the mind on the body. Factors such as the impact of social isolation and stressful life events on health or the placebo effect cannot be explained using the traditional medical model. In every controlled trial, a percentage of people respond physiologically to an inert substance. The magnitude of the placebo effect varies in every study, but it actually approaches 100% in some instances. In a *New England Journal of Medicine* paper aimed at debunking placebos, Hrobjartsson and Gotzsche still found that placebos had a beneficial effect on pain in 27 studies.[35] In an accompanying editorial in that same publication, Dr. John Bailar, Professor Emeritus from the University of Chicago, generally supports their conclusions although he does admit that he feels their recommendations "may be just a bit too sweeping."[36] We believe that these authors are all missing the point. The difference between treatment and healing has to come from within. The mind, as an organ that processes information (beliefs), interacts with the body by producing chemical changes that initiate chain reactions. It seems that these reactions actually determine both our physical and mental health.[37] As Thomas Kuhn has pointed out in *The Structure of Scientific Revolutions*, when a sufficient number of anomalous pieces of information do not fit a particular scientific paradigm, a major conceptual shift must occur.[38]

Perhaps the most important factor to consider in applying the new and more effective medical model is the enhanced practitioner-patient relationship. The role of the practitioner is increasingly to mobilize the patient's own healing power. Norman Cousins underscores the effectiveness of having confidence in the body's recovery potential, involvement in the treatment, and a sense of partnership with the physician as making a major contribution to creating the physiological healing response.[39]

Developing an Integrated (holistic) Approach Based on the Scientific Method

George Engel's conceptualization of the biopsychosocial model presents a relevant paradigm to integrate modern biology and the behavioral sciences in a patient encounter.[40]

Engel states that basic organic building blocks – that is, subatomic particles, atoms, molecules, up through cells, tissues, organs, and organisms – are part of a larger system, including the family, community, and subculture, and on up through the biosphere. He further maintains that these systems are interrelated to the degree that an event impacting on any one component has an effect on all other components. He presents clinical examples, such as the stress-related illness of an electrical engineer, that produce events in a community, such as loss of income, failure of businesses, and outward migration of the population. In this example, he also describes the impact of stress on the engineer's organ systems, with the production of such signs and symptoms as lethargy, pain and nausea.

Building on George Engel's work, McWhinney was perhaps the first to propose that the new paradigm of medicine incorporate the following concepts:

1. paying more attention to health promotion and disease prevention
2. keeping separate disease categories but recognizing the effects of their interactions and patients' disease susceptibility
3. focusing more attention on non-organic factors such as environmental and relationship characteristics when determining the etiology of disease
4. recognizing the physician's role in mobilizing the patient's own healing powers
5. the need for physicians to develop advanced communication skills in order to diagnose and treat patients (rather than diseases)
6. the need to elicit the meaning of the illness to the patient
7. integrating the body, mind and spirit.[41]

Let us look at what might be required to put all these factors into practice.

THE PSYCHOTHERAPEUTIC QUALIFICATIONS OF THE PRIMARY CARE PRACTITIONER

Are primary care practitioners really qualified and competent to integrate body, mind and spirit? Specifically can they handle emotional problems? The good news is that patients think they are. An impressive literature shows that patients clearly consider these clinicians to be their primary source of mental health care.[42,43] A comprehensive study found that patients with psychosocial problems confided in their primary care practitioner more often than any other type of professional. The types of problems included depression, anxiety, bereavement, and marital conflicts, problems with children, and other practical problems, as well as coping with chronic illness. Nearly all the patients (95%) reported that the contact was helpful.[44] Now the bad news! Many practitioners do not know that they are qualified and that they have the skills to be therapeutic; therefore, they do not make the simple interventions that can be highly effective. They often do not even ascertain that there is a problem. Studies have shown that although almost 60% of mental health care is provided in primary care settings, primary care providers fail to recognize up to two thirds of the emotional disorders manifested by their patients.[45] In one study, only 19% of patients who visited primary care providers had their anxiety or depression identified and appropriately treated.[46] More recent studies continue to report that psychiatric disorders are common and that their recognition and treatment remains woefully inadequate with primary practitioners recognizing only about 33% of mental disorders presenting.[47]

Instruments have been developed to alleviate these problems, but they are rarely used routinely with all patients.[48] It is critical to increase the probability of identifying a much greater proportion of these problems and making sure that they are adequately treated.

The Patient's Perspective

Patients do talk to their primary care practitioners about their personal problems. Sometimes they are disappointed when the practitioner, after listening for a while, cuts them off without any acknowledgment or resolution. In our experience physicians receiving training in family medicine frequently do not know what to say next or believe that enough time has been spent listening. So, after having spent some time letting the patient ventilate and nodding at seemingly appropriate places, they return abruptly to the physical symptoms, the "safe" biomedical arena. In spite of this, many patients report feeling better after talking to their doctor, who may not even be aware of the therapeutic process in the interaction or of its impact on the patient.

David Spiegel writing an editorial entitled "Healing Words" in the *Journal of the American Medical Association* in 1999 points out how traditional medicine has focused on the pathophysiology of disease and has ignored the psychophysiological reactions to disease processes. His final comment on the state of current research ends with ". . . it is not simply mind over matter, but it is clear that mind matters."[49] This leads to important clinical questions like: "How do we best impact patients' minds?" or "What specifically can we do to be therapeutic?"

HOW TO BE THERAPEUTIC

So what are the characteristics of a therapeutic relationship? Let us look at a few of the more obvious factors.

Skills

Every practitioner who knows how to talk with and listen to patients has the basic tools with which to provide psychological support. Essential skills in the medical interview consist of establishing rapport, eliciting information, clarifying the patient's problems, and then communicating the diagnosis and management plan. Talking with patients is primarily a theme-centered conversation, a conversation focused on the patient's concerns that should include relevant social, emotional, economic, and spiritual factors. This is the essence of the patient-centered interview.[50]

Trust

The *sine qua non* of any therapeutic relationship is trust. Without trust, skills might be irrelevant. Recent research confirms that ongoing doctor-patient relationships based on trust are critical for effective care.[51-53] Trust can be regarded as an assessment that a person is both competent to fulfill a promise and sincere in the desire to do so. Patients are able to specify the physician behaviors that are associated with trust.[54] Being caring and comforting and demonstrating competence and good communication are the behaviors most strongly associated with patient trust.[51,52]

Traditionally, trust has also implied a patient's expectation of not being rejected or abandoned. Unfortunately, the current health care delivery system often undermines continuity in relationships.[51,52]

Continuity

In primary care, an assumption is made that the practitioner's commitment to the patient has no defined end point. The relationship is one of continuity, with patients assuming that they belong to the practice which has their records, and that they will be taken care of as their needs arise.[55] In 2002 the American Academy of Pediatrics (AAP) described the concept of a medial home to incorporate, in addition to a central location for archiving the medical records of a child, a system of care with the following characteristics: accessible, continuous, comprehensive, family-centered, coordinated, compassionate, and culturally sensitive care.[56]

Five years later the American Academy of Family Physicians, the American Osteopathic Association and the American College of Physicians incorporated this concept into the development of a set of joint principles that describe a new level of primary care which they called the "Patient-Centered Medical Home" (PCMH). These principles address the medical home partnership through which access is facilitated to specialty care, educational services, out-of-home care, family support, and other public and private community services important to the overall health of the patient.[57]

The PCMH is a model of health care delivery based on an ongoing personal relationship with a physician or other primary care practitioner. This committed personal relationship provides continuous and comprehensive health care. The practitioner is responsible for all of the patient's health care needs to include managing care with other qualified professionals, a responsibility that clearly includes the patients' emotional and mental health needs. It is gratifying that there is finally some movement in the United States toward a model of primary care that is working well in Europe and other parts of the world.

When the practitioner is familiar with the patient's family structure, cultural background, orientation toward health care and already knows something about the patient's personal situation, little time is required to be brought up to date. Continuity in the relationship helps the practitioner anticipate critical transitions in the patient's life so that timely interventions can be made. Even in a group practice, this is the patient's medical home. The records reside there and provide continuity even if a different practitioner is seeing the patient. The patient is not at risk of abandonment or rejection.

Providing Support and Comfort

Competent adults are capable of taking care of themselves and of others who are dependent. However, when feeling down, besieged, or overwhelmed by physical or mental stressors, as will be discussed in the next chapter, everyone experiences a need to be supported, nurtured, and comforted. Adults, children, practitioners, and patients are all vulnerable to the same conditions. The more our resources feel depleted by virtue of the forces impinging on us, the more dependent we become. When this happens, support from others becomes an emergent need. Patients generally feel better after a medical visit. Getting a prescription for medicine, the written excuse or a filled out form, may be a symbol for the sustenance that the patient seeks, but the caring can be entirely in the process.

THE ISSUE OF POWER

Although practitioners are generally very aware of their power to affect life and death by the medical decisions they make, especially in the hospital setting, not having been exposed to the literature on social power, few are aware of their impressive potential to influence patients' attitudes and behavior.

What Is Social Power?

Social power has been defined as the potential that one person has to change the beliefs, attitudes, or behavior of another person.[58] Changing a patient's beliefs, attitudes, or behavior is the essence of the therapeutic intervention. In general, power can be defined as the potential or ability to satisfy needs. If we can satisfy our own needs, we have personal power. If we are in a position to satisfy other peoples' needs or if they assume that we can satisfy their needs, they give us power, and allow us to influence their behavior, thoughts, and feelings. It is useful to look at the power base that operates in the practitioner-patient relationship.

TYPES OF SOCIAL POWER

In the 1950s, French and Raven analyzed a large body of empirical research on social power, that is, the psychological changes induced in a relationship between an influencer and an object. Their original formulation distinguished five specific types of power: reward, coercive, referent, legitimate, and expert. Multiple types of power in a relationship were seen to increase the power base. In their later expanded model, they added information as a separate source of social power and examined variables such as the motivation of the influencer, values, and norms, as well as the positive and negative effects of power bases.[59] In our view, access to (medical) information is part of expert power and not a separate category and we assume that practitioners are motivated to use their power for the benefit of the patient. So it is useful to examine the five original sources of social power since the primary care practitioner generally has all of them in relation to a patient.

Reward Power

The first type of social power, reward power, consists of the ability or resources to provide symbolic or material rewards: giving people what they want or need. In a practitioner-patient interaction, this might be attention, time, prescriptions, reassurance, approval, or advice. It can mean responding favorably to requests for information, medication, tests, procedures, or filling out administrative forms, that is, providing relief from disease, pain, or anxiety.

Coercive Power

Coercive power depends on the ability to respond to a person's behavior in punitive ways, i.e., to create negative or uncomfortable consequences. Coercive power works well in situations where one has a captive audience, but undermines the quality of relationships. Coercive power is omnipresent in the practitioner's potential for expressing disapproval, denying requests, prescribing aversive protocols, refusing to see patients or answer phone calls, and withholding permission for desired activities. Behavior that changes in response to coercion generally reverts back to its natural form when supervision is removed.

The ineffectiveness of coercive power, in the absence of supervision, may well account for the dismal rate of patient compliance with medication regimens, especially when patients are dissatisfied with their relationships with their practitioners.[60,61]

Referent Power

The most potent social power, referent power, is defined by a person's desire to identify with an attractive power source. The advertising industry spends billions of dollars capitalizing on the effectiveness of referent power, brandishing portraits of the most popular current sports hero in advertisements promoting everything from cereal to sneakers or automobiles.[62] The positive feelings generated by the thought of associating oneself with a person or a group, connected by shared beliefs, are the most powerful and lasting way to influence a person.[63] Attitude or behavior change induced by referent power becomes internalized and self-maintaining quite rapidly. People want to be like the role model, mentor, hero, or "admired other" any way they can. They want to use the same products, engage in the same behaviors, and have the same opinions. It feels good. It makes them feel connected. That feeling further reinforces the power of the revered object.

Referent power can help ensure treatment adherence in the outpatient setting. When the patient admires the practitioner and wants to both be like and be liked by the practitioner, cooperation is rewarding. Patients feel virtuous and competent when following the doctor's orders. Telling other people that "my doctor says I'm doing well," "understands that I feel awful," or "wants to see me again in a couple of weeks" makes patients feel good.

Legitimate Power

Legitimate power derives from perceptions that another person has an institutionalized right to exert influence. When a patient initiates a consultation, legitimate power is attributed to the practitioner. By contracting to pay for advice given, whether directly or through a third party, patients acknowledge the legitimacy of the practitioner's right to give instructions and their obligation to cooperate.

The more legitimate the power is perceived to be, the less resistance there is to the influence exerted. However, when patients have ambivalent feelings toward authority growing out of a history of conflicts with coercive or overly demanding authority figures (e.g., parents, teachers, employers), they may challenge the authority of the practitioner. Since many patients have some problems with authority, adherence to treatment recommendations is not always ensured, regardless of the contractual relationship. In subsequent chapters we will discuss ways to avoid power struggles smoothly.

Expert Power

Unquestionably, patients accept the practitioner as an expert in medical matters, including access to relevant information, and hence are open to being influenced. Even with the plethora of information available directly to patients on the internet, the practitioner's word on physical, psychological or social matters is rarely questioned. Regardless of the actual level of the practitioner's knowledge, most patients attribute global expert power to the practitioner.

Facilitating Change

The more under stress or unsure about an issue a person feels, the more open that person is to help and suggestion. The more difficult the matter is to understand, the more persuasive the arguments of an expert are found to be. Conversely, when people hold firm beliefs or simplistic understandings, these must first be explored and validated before counter arguments can be effective. Motivational interviewing capitalizes on this phenomenom.[64] The interview helps the patient to sort out the positive and negative consequences of either changing or not changing a particular behavior. In this case, influence is applied through a process, rather than imposing a demand or issuing an edict for change.

People change their beliefs and also their behavior when they are convinced by information that, although different from their previous understanding, presents a convincing picture based on the qualifications of the source providing the new information. But people change only when they feel safe to do so and when they are ready.

Eliciting the Context of the Visit

When a patient presents to a primary care practitioner, it is important to ascertain the reason that the patient has chosen this time to seek medical attention. It is, however, essential that this process does not consume inordinate amounts of time. We have devised a simple and efficient protocol to explore the psychosocial context that has very specific, limited goals:

1. raising the patient's awareness of the concomitant events that might be affecting his or her health status
2. focusing the patient on the emotional state that is being experienced
3. guiding the patient into specifying one aspect of the problem that is particularly troubling
4. ascertaining the manner in which the patient is handling the experienced stress
5. using active listening and providing an empathic response, to make the patient feel validated.

We ask four basic questions: What is going on? How do you feel about it? What troubles you the most? How are you handling that? We then paraphrase our understanding of the problem, and state that the patient is handling it as well as

12

can be expected under the circumstances. Finishing with this type of empathic response is crucial. As pointed out previously, no response or an abrupt change of topic may leave a patient feeling dissatisfied, even when the practitioner has spent time and given the patient the opportunity to ventilate about a problem. Any time a patient expresses concerns about some issue, the practitioner *must* respond empathically. We suggest that whenever a practitioner is at a loss for words after being presented with some complicated or painful problem, the automatic reply "That must be very difficult (or hard, painful, tiring, or discouraging) for you" is generally appropriate. This type of confirmation, coming from a powerful, attractive, knowledgeable source, makes the patient feel affirmed. Although the situation is tough, at least the response is reasonable. The patient feels better, not as subjectively out of control. Perhaps he or she is not as incompetent, worthless, or helpless as had been imagined; and perhaps it is not true that "nobody cares," since the clinician obviously cares. Hope is rekindled. The patient is no longer demoralized. Tolerance for symptoms will be enhanced, and the healing capacity of the body will be facilitated.[65,66]

Often patients will go into great detail about their situations. Paraphrasing the patient's concerns demonstrates attentive listening and will reduce the amount of detail and repetition in the patient's story. When the practitioner interjects that the situation obviously is difficult and he or she looks forward to hearing the outcome in follow-up, this allows the patient to move on. These easy-to-learn techniques provide psychological support and hence address the emotional component of the patient's problems. Primary care practitioners are both qualified and able to manage these issues since they have both the skills and the opportunity to make effective therapeutic interventions.

A Brief Clinical Example

A 24-year-old woman visited the office, complaining of a sore throat and a mild earache that she had had for 10 days. The chart showed that there had been several previous visits for minor complaints and some evidence of mild postpartum depression. Her youngest child was currently 12 months old. There were two older children in the home. Questioning elicited no particular acute stress, just a general lack of enthusiasm. When asked about the progress of the baby, the patient brightened somewhat. The practitioner then suggested that taking care of an active one-year-old, especially at a busy time of the year and when she wasn't feeling well herself, must be very difficult. The patient gave a deep sigh, "Oh, how I wish that there was someone to take care of me." The practitioner responded, "I can understand that. It must be hard to constantly have to be in the role of nurturing Mom." He put his hand on her shoulder and gently guided her to the exam table. She smiled and relaxed. During the course of the exam he asked her to think about what *she* could do to carve out short periods of time to take care of herself.

This simple interaction did not solve the patient's problems or cure her "mild depression." However, as a result of the interaction, the patient obviously felt better, as shown by her affect. We assume that she interpreted the practitioner's comments as indicating that her response to her problems was reasonable and that therefore she was seen as a reasonable person. This lifted her spirits and her self-esteem. She was also empowered by permission to plan for her own needs as well as those of her children.

DIFFERENCES IN APPROACH BETWEEN PRIMARY CARE PRACTITIONERS AND MENTAL HEALTH SPECIALISTS

Obviously there are major differences in both process and outcome between therapeutic interventions that are provided by primary care practitioners and specialty treatment by psychiatrists or other mental health professionals. In primary care we provide symptomatic treatment without extensive psychiatric evaluation or diagnosis. Physicians who are psychiatrists are specialists trained to treat people who are seriously ill and may well be wasting their talents treating those who are less disturbed. Primary care practitioners treat a different patient population. Every case of chest pain does not warrant referral to a cardiologist. Even when a mental health referral is indicated, whether to a psychiatrist or other mental health professional for talk therapy, many patients experience serious impediments to receiving treatment. Some of these obstacles are financial, some are logistical, and some have to do with the patient's reluctance to pursue treatment because they are not comfortable with the notion that they need it.[67] Better outcomes can be expected when mental health services are directly integrated into primary care.[68]

Normalizing Emotional Histories

Psychiatrists are trained to look for psychopathological conditions and to describe and classify the observed phenomena according to the appropriate category in the latest edition of the American Psychiatric Association's *Diagnostic and Statistical Manual of Mental Disorders*. Primary care practitioners see a different spectrum of patients presenting with undifferentiated problems. Although in psychiatry and other mental health disciplines the process of making a diagnosis is part of the treatment, this activity may intimidate patients who are commonly referred because of stress or relationship problems.[69]

Regardless of other presenting problems, we believe it is part of the primary care practitioner's task to look for and address psychological distress experienced by patients. If the emotional component is left untreated, patients are apt to attempt to relieve their suffering by repeated and often inappropriate use of medical services.[70] However, psychosocial information should be gathered in a therapeutic manner, providing support rather than generating additional stress for the patient.

Collaborative mental health care, ideally with counselors actually located

14

within the primary care setting, is a recent option.[71,72] Studies of psychosocial treatments in primary care provide support for the effectiveness of this type of intervention.[69]

Referrals for Mental Health Treatment Are Often Not Completed

Patients are often reluctant to admit that they need psychiatric treatment.[67,73] The idea of defining themselves as mental patients is an impediment to seeking help because of the stigma that may be attached. Even when referrals are made, patients often do not follow through.[74] Studies show that somewhere between 15% and 75% of patients who are referred for psychiatric treatment fail to keep initial appointments.[75] Those patients who are most resistant to completing referrals also make more medical visits, generally presenting with difficult-to-explain somatic symptoms.[76] In one study of children referred for mental health treatment because of psychosocial problems only 30.5% of the referred patients saw a mental health provider more than once during the six-month follow-up period.[77] There is some evidence that even a single session of psychotherapy can be very effective.[78] However, when patients are referred and it is not their idea, not only is the dropout rate high, but as Bowden and his colleagues found, about half of the patients dropping out may feel worse than when starting treatment.[79] Even when wanting to make a referral, practitioners often face severe challenges in arranging for mental health services for their patients.[80,81] Therefore, practitioners need to feel comfortable providing interim treatment.

In our view, some very important and effective therapeutic interventions can be made directly by primary care practitioners. Furthermore, these interventions are different in several respects from those generally employed by psychiatrists. Let us look at some of these differences.

Treatment of Symptoms Without Pathological Labeling

The first major difference is that the primary care practitioner can treat the patient's emotional reaction to whatever environmental stress is being experienced without labeling the patient as a mental patient. The patient receives the help that is asked for (relief of symptoms) and does not have to deal with the idea of seeing a "shrink." Actually, it has been our experience that after working with the primary care practitioner on the emotional overlay attached to various physical problems, patients will often request a referral to a mental health practitioner in order to extend their work of self-exploration. One of the most beneficial aspects of the therapeutic relationship with the primary care practitioner may be to prepare the patient for needed in-depth mental health treatment.[82]

When patients start to experience the benefits of increased levels of personal awareness and control, they often overcome the reluctance to engage in psychological or psychiatric treatment. However, the timely intervention by the primary care practitioner may restore normal functioning or even improve normal functioning to such an extent that the patient does not need further treatment.

Small Doses of Therapy at a Time

The second major difference between therapeutic interventions provided by the primary care practitioner and traditional psychiatric treatment is that the patient receives small doses of psychotherapy as a part of the regular medical visit. Every part of the interaction with the practitioner is potentially therapeutic. We have gone to great lengths to point out the amount of social power that is attributed to practitioners. Because of this power, the personal exchanges, both verbal and nonverbal, that occur during the normal office visit can have tremendous impact on the patient. Since each of us has an assumptive map, a mental representation of ourselves and our world based on personal history as we have recorded it (our story), our perception of ourselves can be influenced by how we see ourselves treated by significant others with whom we come in contact.[83] If our story line has been that we are not at all important and that no one cares about us and then, over time, we are repeatedly treated well by an important person, after some initial discounting and disbelief, we may change our assumptive map and edit our story. As the weight of evidence countering our preconceived notions about ourselves increases, we are able to make a change in our self-image. This may actually take the form of a paradigm shift as explained earlier.

Small repeated doses of therapeutic messages may actually be more effective, in terms of being heard, believed, and integrated, than a large dose at one time, which may be more difficult to swallow and to assimilate. People learn by repetition over a period of time but only when it is psychologically safe for them to do so and when they are ready to learn.

The Patient Does Not Feel Rejected

The third major factor to be considered in providing psychological treatment personally rather than making a referral, even when appropriate, is that often the patient may interpret the referral as rejection. If the patient feels comfortable with and trusts the practitioner, there is a natural reluctance to start over with someone new. Being referred may also play into the self-deprecating pathological view of the patient. When a patient's self-esteem is low and the practitioner responds by pushing the patient away, sending the patient to see someone else, this may confirm the patient's view that "no one can or wants to help." The patient may feel that there is little use in even trying. In contrast, the practitioner's commitment to helping the patient is interpreted as an indication that the situation may be far less serious than the patient has assumed and that the patient is more worthy of help. Naturally, there will be times that a referral must be made because the practitioner feels overwhelmed. We will discuss this in a subsequent section.

The Body and the Mind Are Not Separated

Especially in the case of psychosomatic illness, rather than exploring all the organic elements before trying to convince the patient that psychological treatment is indicated, we treat physical and psychological components of the problem concurrently. This may, over time, convince patients of the connection between their physical symptoms and the stressors in their lives. Writing in the *New England Journal of Medicine* about functional gastrointestinal disorders, J.E. Lennard-Jones pointed out the importance of making the psychosocial history part of the initial inquiry "because a sudden interest in possible psychological factors after investigations have given normal results can arouse hostility in the patient."[84] Patients with psychosomatic problems who are referred to psychiatrists after a full exploration of their somatic complaints are notorious for seeking further medical opinions and being refractory to psychiatric treatment.[85] In addition, the focus on purely biomedical problems is not necessarily benign. Harrington has pointed out that practitioners often unwittingly precipitate or perpetuate patients' emotional illness. "Every psychiatrist sees patients who have been in the hands of three or four different specialists, all of whom are said to have told the patient something different. Such patients are hard to treat because they have lost faith."[86]

When the psychiatrist puts emphasis exclusively on the mind instead of the body, this reverse split is no more productive than looking for pathological conditions only in tissues and organs. Specialization often fragments patients' care, when fragmentation in the fabric of our society, or fragmentation in the structure of the patient's family or work situation, might be precipitating the illness in the first place.

Knowledge of the Family

Since the primary care practitioner generally knows the circumstances of a patient's family constellation and has had personal contact with the cast of characters involved, it becomes easier to empathize with the patient's experience. "Yes, I know Mary can be difficult to deal with. What can you do to make her feel more secure?" can be a powerful intervention, coming from someone who has had dealings with Mary. The patient already trusts the practitioner, whereas the psychiatrist is an unknown individual who is suspect simply because of being cast in the role of psychiatrist, that is, evaluator and analyst.

Thus the major difference in approach is that the primary care practitioner, in contrast to the mental health specialist, helps the patient make a more comfortable adaptation to the existing environment, without getting into the technicalities of the patient's personality structure, specific defense mechanisms, or even family dynamics, since these are difficult to change (except in a crisis). Instead, the practitioner focuses on the reaction that the person is experiencing to perceived stress of the moment. This reaction may be anxiety, depression, and/or any number of physical complaints. By providing support and focusing the patient on constructive action, the practitioner helps to enhance the patient's self-esteem and enables the patient to function at a more productive level.

SUMMARY

Recognizing the interrelationship between physical and psychological health, the true inseparability of the psyche and the soma, and the tension between the scientific method and the patient's needs, the clinician is urged to focus on the process of the practitioner-patient relationship. There is a need to incorporate the insights from George Engel's biopsychosocial model, in order to develop communication skills that will help foster a therapeutic encounter to support the inherent strength of the patient and promote his or her own healing powers. The true healing skills are those of communication and caring. Primary care practitioners have the necessary interviewing skills to establish relationships of trust, continuity, comfort, and support for their patients as a base for making therapeutic interventions.

Social power is defined as the potential to influence the beliefs, attitudes, or behavior of another person. Being powerful, attractive, and credible sources of information, practitioners have the potential to influence patients' behavior and effect permanent attitude change. The power attributed to practitioners can be used with awareness, in the service of making patients feel better about themselves and their world. By establishing the context of the patient's visit and providing an empathic response, the practitioner can identify and help to mitigate the patient's distress.

The primary care practitioner's commitment to the patient is always to provide care within the scope of the practitioner's expertise. We recommend treating the patient's symptoms within the context of the medical problems presented. By refraining from analyzing or explaining the origin of behavior, while helping the patient manage reactions to situations, the practitioner's approach is different from that of a traditional psychiatrist or other mental health professional. Patients are not required to define themselves as mental patients when treated by their primary care practitioner. Symptoms can be treated without pathological labels. Small doses of therapy at a time may prove quite effective. Referrals for collaborative care can be made when appropriate. In the meantime, the patient does not feel rejected, and the body and mind are not separated.

References

1. Holman EA, Silver RC, Poulin M, *et al.* Terrorism, acute stress, and cardiovascular health: a 3-year national study following the September 11th attacks. *Arch Gen Psychiatry.* 2008; **65**(1): 73–80.
2. Norquist GS, Regier DA. The epidemiology of psychiatric disorders and the de facto mental health care system. *Ann Rev Med.* 1996; **47**: 473–9.
3. Wang PS, Lane M, Olfson M, *et al.* Twelve-month use of mental health services in

the United States: results from the National Comorbidity Survey Replication. *Arch Gen Psychiatry.* 2005; **62**: 629–40.

4. Eisenberg L. Treating depression and anxiety in primary care: closing the gap between knowledge and practice. *N Eng J Med.* 1992; **326**(16): 1080–4.

5. Roberts L, Battaglia J, Epstein, R. Frontier ethics: mental health care needs and ethical dilemmas in rural communities. *Psychiatr Serv.* 1999; **50**(4): 497–503.

6. Engel GL. The clinical application of the biopsychosocial model. *Am J Psychia.* 1980; **137**: 535–44, p. 536.

7. Barsky AJ. Hidden reasons some patients visit doctors. *Ann Int Med.* 1981; **94**(1): 492–8.

8. Dantzer R. Stress and disease: a psychobiological perspective. *Ann Behav Med.* 1991; **13**: 205–10.

9. MacDonald G, Leary MR. Why does social exclusion hurt? The relationship between social and physical pain. *Psych Bull.* 2005; **131**(2): 202–3.

10. Eisenberger NI, Lieberman MD, Williams KD. Does rejection hurt? An fMRI study of social exclusion. *Science.* 2003; **302**(5643): 290–2.

11. Eng PM, Rimm EB, Fitzmaurice G, *et al.* Social ties and change in social ties in relation to subsequent total and cause-specific mortality and coronary heart disease incidence in men. *Am J Epidemiol.* 2002; **155**(8): 700–9.

12. Martin BI, Deyo RA, Mirza SK, *et al.* Expenditures and health status among adults with back and neck problems. *JAMA.* 2008; **299**(6): 656–4.

13. Schiltenwolf M, Buchner M, Heindl B, *et al.* Comparison of a biopsychosocial therapy (BT) with a conventional biomedical therapy (MT) of subacute low back pain in the first episode of sick leave: a randomized controlled trial. *EurSpine.* 2006; **15**(7): 1083–92.

14. Greer S, Morris T, Pettingale KW. Psychological response to breast cancer: effects on outcome. *Lancet.* 1979; **13**: 785–7.

15. Spiegel D, Bloom J, Kraemer HC, *et al.* Effect of psychosocial treatment on the survival of patients with metastatic breast cancer. *Lancet.* 1989; **2**: 888–91.

16. Garsen B, Goodkin K. On the role of immunological factors as mediators between psychosocial factors and cancer progression. *Psych Res.* 1999; **85**: 51–61.

17. Watson M, Homewood J, Haviland J, *et al.* Influence of psychological response on breast cancer survival: 10-year follow-up of a population-based cohort. *Eur J Cancer.* 2005; **41**(12): 1710–14.

18. Bartrop, R, Lazarus L, Luckherst E, *et al.* Depressed lymphocyte function after bereavement. *Lancet.* 1977; **1**: 834–6.

19. Schleifer SJ, Keller SE, Camerino M, *et al.* Suppression of lymphocyte stimulation following bereavement. *JAMA.* 1983; **250**: 374–7.

20. Kiecolt-Glaser JK, McGuire L, Robles TF, *et al.* Emotions, morbidity, and mortality: new perspectives from psychoneuroimmunology. *Ann Rev Psychol.* 2002; **53**: 83–107.

21. Ader R, Kelley KW. A global view of twenty years of brain, behavior, and immunity. *Brain Behav Immunol.* 2007; **21**(1): 20–2.

22. Irwin MR. Human psychoneuroimmunology: 20 years of discovery. *Brain Behav Immunol.* 2008; **22**(2): 129–39.

23. Spence MJ, Moss-Morris R. The cognitive behavioural model of irritable bowel syndrome: a prospective investigation of patients with gastroenteritis. *Gut.* 2007; **56**(8): 1066–71.

24. Wiesli P, Schmid C, Kerwer O, *et al.* Acute psychological stress affects glucose concentrations in patients with type 1 diabetes following food intake but not in the fasting state. *Diabetes Care.* 2005; **28**(8): 1910–15.
25. Karling P, Norrback KF, Adolfsson R, *et al.* Gastrointestinal symptoms are associated with hypothalamic-pituitary-adrenal axis suppression in healthy individuals. *Scand J Gastroenterol.* 2007; **42**(11): 1294–301.
26. Smith TW. Hostility and health: current status of a psychosomatic hypothesis. *Health Psych.* 1992; **11**: 139–50.
27. Wassertheil-Smoller S, Applegate WB, Berge K. Change in depression as a precursor of cardiovascular events. *Arch Int Med.* 1996; **156**: 553–61.
28. Shen BJ, Avivi YE, Todaro JF, *et al.* Anxiety characteristics independently and prospectively predict myocardial infarction in men: the unique contribution of anxiety among psychologic factors. *J Am Coll Cardiol.* 2008; **51**(2): 113–19.
29. Shipley BA, Weiss A, Der G, *et al.* Neuroticism, extraversion, and mortality in the UK Health and Lifestyle Survey: a 21-year prospective cohort study. *Psychosom Med.* 2007; **69**(9): 923–31.
30. Tennant C. Life stress, social support and coronary heart disease. *Aust N Z J Psychiatry.* 1999; **33**: 636–41.
31. Smith DF. Negative emotions and coronary heart disease: causally related or merely coexistent? A review. *Scand J Psychol.* 2001; **42**: 57–69.
32. Thurston RC, Kubzansky LD. Multiple sources of psychosocial disadvantage and risk of coronary heart disease. *Psychosom Med.* 2007; **69**(8): 748–55.
33. McWhinney I. *A Textbook of Family Medicine.* (2nd ed.). New York: Oxford University Press; 1997. p. 50.
34. Kroenke K, Mangelsdorff AD. Common symptoms in ambulatory care: incidence, evaluation, therapy, and outcome. *Am J Med.* 1989; **86**(3): 262–6.
35. Hrobjartsson A, Gotzsche PC. Is the placebo powerless? *N Eng J Med.* 2001; **344**: 1594–602.
36. Bailar JC. The powerful placebo and the wizard of oz. *N Eng J Med.* 2001; **344**: 1630–2.
37. McEwen BS, Wingfield JC. The concept of allostasis in biology and biomedicine. *Horm Behav.* 2003; **43**: 2–15.
38. Kuhn TS. *The Structure of Scientific Revolutions.* Chicago: University of Chicago Press; 1962.
39. Cousins N. *The Healing Heart: antidotes to panic and helplessness.* New York: Norton; 1983. pp. 12–13.
40. Engel GL. The need for a new medical model: a challenge for biomedicine. *Science.* 1977; **196**: 129–36.
41. McWhinney I. *Time, change and the physician.* Plenary Address to the Society of Teachers of Family Medicine. 16th Annual Spring Conference, May 1983.
42. Üstun TB, Von Korff M. Primary mental health services: access and provision of care. In: Üstun TB, Sartorius N, (eds.) *Mental Illness in General Health Care: an international study.* New York: Wiley; 1995.
43. Kessler RC, Merikangas KR, Wang PS. Prevalence, comorbidity, and service utilization for mood disorders in the United States at the beginning of the twenty-first century. *Ann Rev Clin Psychol.* 2007; **3**(1): 137–58.
44. Corney RH. A survey of professional help sought by patients for psychosocial problems. *Brit J Gen Pract.* 1990; **40**: 365–8.

45. Kessler D, Lloyd K, Lewis G, *et al.* Cross-sectional study of symptom attribution and recognition of depression and anxiety in primary care. *BMJ.* 1999; **318**: 436–9.

46. Young AS, Klap R, Sherbourne C, *et al.* The quality of care for depressive and anxiety disorders in the United States. *Arch Gen Psychiatry.* 2001; **58**: 55–61.

47. Jackson JL, Passamonti M, Kroenke K. Outcome and impact of mental disorders in primary care at 5 years. *Psychosom Med.* 2007; **69**(3): 270–6.

48. Spitzer RL, Kroenke K, Linzer FV. Health-related quality of life in primary care patients with mental disorders: results from the PRIME-MD 1000 Study. *JAMA.*1995; **274**: 1511–17.

49. Spiegel D. Healing words: emotional expression and disease outcome. *JAMA.* 1999; **281**(14): 1328–9.

50. Brown JB, Stewart MA, McCracken MC, *et al.* The patient centered clinical method: definition and application. *Fam Pract.*1986; **3**: 75–9.

51. Murphy J, Chang H, Montgomery JE, *et al.* The quality of physician-patient relationships: patients' experiences 1996-1999. *J Fam Pract.* 2001; **50**(2): 123–9.

52. Safran DG, Montgomery JA, Chang H, *et al.* Switching doctors: predictors of voluntary disenrollment from a primary physician's practice. *J Fam Prac.* 2001; **50**(2): 130–6.

53. Berry LL, Parish JT, Janakiraman R, *et al.* Patients' commitment to their primary physician and why it matters. *Ann Fam Med.* 2008; **6**(1): 6–13.

54. Thom DH, Stanford Trust Study Physicians. Physician behaviors that predict trust. *J Fam Pract.* 2001; **50**(4): 323–8.

55. McWhinney IR. *A Textbook of Family Medicine.* New York: Oxford University Press; 1989.

56. Sia C, Tonniges TF, Osterhus E, *et al.* History of the medical home concept. *Pediatrics.* 2004; **113**(5 Suppl.): 1473–8.

57. American Academy of Family Physicians, American Academy of Pediatrics, American College of Physicians, American Osteopathic Association. *Joint Principles of the Patient-centered Medical Home.* March 2007. Available at: www. medicalhomeinfo.org/Joint%20Statement.pdf (accessed 28 January 2007).

58. French JPR Jr., Raven BH. The bases of social power. In: Cartwright D, Zander A, (eds.) *Group Dynamics: research and theory.* 3rd ed. New York: Harper & Row; 1968.

59. Raven BA. Power/interaction model of interpersonal influence: French and Raven thirty years later. *J Soc Behav Pers.* 1992; **7**(2): 217–44.

60. Van Dulmen S, Sluijs E, Van Dijk L, *et al.* Patient adherence to medical treatment: a review of reviews. *BMC Health Serv Res.* 2007; **17**(7): 55.

61. Krueger KP, Felkey BG, Berger BA. Improving adherence and persistence: a review and assessment of interventions and description of steps toward a national adherence initiative. *J Am Pharm Ass.* 2003; **43**(6): 668–78.

62. Kukcevich D. Forbes faces: Tiger Woods. *Forbes;* Nov 14, 2000. www.forbes.com (accessed 12 June 2001).

63. Kelman HC. Compliance, identification and internalization: three processes of attitude change. *J Conflict Res.* 1958; **2**: 51–60.

64. Rollnick S, Miller WR. What is motivational interviewing? *Behav Cog Psychother.* 1995; **23**: 325–39.

65. Cassel J. The contribution of the social environment to host resistance. *Am J Epidemiol.* 1976; **104**: 107–23.

66. Cohen S. Social relationships and health. *Am Psychol.* 2004; **60**: 676–84.
67. Mechanic D. Barriers to help-seeking, detection, and adequate treatment for anxiety and mood disorders: implications for health care policy. *J Clin Psychiatry.* 2007; **68**(Suppl. 2): 20–6.
68. Fisher L, Ransom DC. Developing a strategy for managing behavioral health care within the context of primary care. *Arch Fam Med.* 1997: **6**: 324–33.
69. Hemmings A. A systemic review of the effectiveness of brief psychological therapies in primary health care. *Fam Syst Health.* 2000; **18**: 279–313.
70. Goldberg DP, Bridges K. Somatic presentations of psychiatric illness in primary care setting. *J Psychosom Res.* 1988; **32**: 137–44.
71. Lorenz AD, Mauksch LB, Gawinski BA. Models of collaboration. *Prim Care.* 1999; **26**: 401–10.
72. Jenkins GC. Collaborative care in the United Kingdom. *Prim Care.* 1999; **26**: 411–22.
73. Ben-Noun L. Characterization of patients refusing professional psychiatric treatment in a primary care clinic. *Israeli J Psychia Rel Sci.* 1996; **33**(3): 167–74.
74. Carpenter PJ, Morrow GR, Del Gaudio AC, *et al.* Who keeps the first outpatient appointment? *Am J Psychiatry.* 1981; **138**: 102–5.
75. Dobscha SK, Delucchi K, Yound ML. Adherence with referrals for outpatient follow-up from a VA psychiatric emergency room. *Com Ment Health J.* 1999; **35**(5): 451–8.
76. Olfson M. Primary care patients who refuse specialized mental health services. *Arch Int Med.* 1991; **151**: 129–32.
77. Rushton J, Bruckman D, Kelleher K. Primary care referral of children with psychosocial problems. *Arch Pediatr Adolesc Med.* 2002; **156**: 592–8.
78. Rossi A, Amaddeo F, Sandri M, *et al.* What happens to patients seen only once by psychiatric services? Findings from a follow-up study. *Psychia Res.* 2008; **157**(1-3): 53–65.
79. Bowden CL, Schoenfeld LS, Adams RL. A correlation between dropout status and improvement in a psychiatric clinic. *Hosp Community Psychiatry.* 1980; **31**: 192–5.
80. Trude S, Stoddard JJ. Referral gridlock; primary care physicians and mental health services. *J Gen Intern Med.* 2003; **18**(6): 442–9.
81. Walders N, Childs GE, Comer D, *et al.* Barriers to mental health referral from pediatric primary care settings. *Am J Manag Care.* 2003; **9**(10): 677–83.
82. Larson DL, Nguyen TD, Green RS, *et al.* Enhancing the utilization of outpatient mental health services. *Com Mental Health J.* 1983; **19**: 305–20.
83. Bandler R, Grinder J. *The Structure of Magic. I. A Book About Language and Therapy.* Palo Alto, CA: Science and Behavior Books; 1975.
84. Lennard-Jones JE. Functional gastrointestinal disorders. *New Eng J Med.* 1983; **308**: 431–5.
85. Oyama O, Paltoo C, Greengold J. Somatoform disorders. *Am Fam Physician.* 2007; **76**(9): 1333–8.
86. Harrington JA. Some principles of psychotherapy in general practice. *Lancet.* 1957; **1**: 799–801.

CHAPTER 2

Patients, Stress, and the Office Visit

According to a national survey released by the American Psychological Society (APA) in late 2007, one-third of Americans are living with extreme stress and nearly half of Americans (48%) report that their stress has increased over the past five years. This stress is contributing to health problems, damaging relationships and leading to lost productivity at work.[1] As many as 77% of people report experiencing physical symptoms as well as psychological symptoms related to their stress in a particular month. Symptoms reported included fatigue, headache, upset stomach, muscle pain, change in appetite, teeth grinding, change in sex drive, and feeling dizzy. Fifty percent of people report symptoms of stress manifesting psychologically as irritability or anger, others report feeling nervous, lack of energy, feeling as though "you could cry" and almost half complain of lying awake at night due to stress.[1] The bottom line for the primary care practitioner is to be aware that when patients come into the office complaining of any of the above conditions, it is important to briefly examine the circumstances of their lives.

The purpose of *The Fifteen Minute Hour* is to present easy interventions you can use to help patients cope with the stress in their lives, positively modify their lifestyles and manage their illnesses more effectively.

STRESS AND ALLOSTATIC LOAD

Hans Selye[2] first defined stress as a non-specific biological mobilization for action required to adapt to change or to respond to a threat. Although this autonomic nervous system reaction is often thought of as a standard process (achieving the physiological readiness for fight or flight) many factors, including personality traits, coping styles, and the availability of social support mediate the relationship between stress and illness.

Recently a new concept has been introduced that we find clinically useful.

23

Bruce McEwen[3] points out that psychological and experiential factors are often powerful activators of the stress response as manifested by hypothalamic/pituitary/adrenal (HPA) axis and autonomic nervous system (ANS) activity. However, he suggests that when dealing with chronic stressors the brain is amazingly resilient and capable of adaptive plasticity. Since stress is defined as an event or events interpreted by the brain as threatening to a person, the *brain* is the key organ involved in precipitating the stress response. Similar to the body's need to maintain homeostasis in relation to temperature, chemicals, and fluid balances, McEwen[3] introduces the concept of "allostasis" referring to the coping mechanisms used to deal with stress to maintain stability and to promote adaptation and coping. There is however, a cost to the body when these mechanisms are used too frequently or not effectively. McEwen[3] refers to this as "allostatic load." Allostatic load refers to the cumulative negative effect, or the price the body pays for being forced to adapt to numerous psychosocial challenges and adverse situations. Allostatic load is determined by the inefficiency of a person's response to stress, or how many challenges an individual experiences. In our later discussions of cognitive behavioral therapy we will show that by encouraging patients to change their interpretations and reactions to stress, they will effectively decrease their "allostatic load" and promote their physical as well as mental health.

SOCIAL SUPPORT

We mentioned earlier that patients' reactions to stress are influenced by many factors including personality traits, coping styles and the availability of social support. Personality traits, by definition, are set patterns, and coping styles vary in effectiveness, but social support is a resource that can be mobilized rapidly by concerned others. The presence of social support minimizes the effect of "allostatic load."

Social support can be understood as a psychological mechanism that provides positive information to help people reassess or redefine perceptions regarding themselves, their situation or the *quality* of their interpersonal relationships. The information may be about the individual, about the relationship or about solutions for a problem. It is the positive quality of social support that aids the individual to develop more positive expectations and subsequently behave in a manner to realize these expectations. Social support appears to have important direct and indirect health effects. Some of the indirect effects of strong social support include healthier coping processes in rheumatoid arthritis patients[4] and greater wellbeing in breast cancer survivors.[5]

Perhaps more compelling are the findings from studies examining the direct effects of social support on health outcomes. For example, maintaining more diverse social networks is associated with greater resistance to the common cold.[6] Conversely, poor social support appears to be an independent risk factor for how acute coronary heart disease events[7] interact with life stressors to increase risk of breast carcinoma.[8] Inadequate social support also predicts poor pregnancy outcomes even after controlling for biomedical risk.[9]

THE STORY AS PERSONAL STEADY STATE

Just as every part of the human organism is involved in maintaining homeostasis, each person strives to maintain a personal/social steady state in relation to other people. Interpretations of subjective experiences of interactions with others are stored in peoples' memories. This recorded information is used to develop expectations for subsequent encounters, becoming part of a person's "story." These stories then continue to affect peoples' behavior, and cause expectations to become self-fulfilling prophecies. In later chapters, we will discuss how to listen to and help people modify their stories.

DETERMINING THE CONTEXT OF THE VISIT

Probably the most important question that any practitioner asks about a patient's visit (other than an acute, life-threatening episode) is "Why is the patient coming now?" Mr. Jones has had a sore throat for two weeks. He denies any fever. He has no cough or other symptoms. His throat is slightly erythematous. What made him decide to come today? He does not seem to be that sick. It would seem that he has felt at least this bad for the past two weeks. So why did he come in now? The best way to find out what Mr. Jones is concerned about is to ask him. "What are you afraid is going on?" It is also important to get some idea of what is going on in his life. What level of stress is he dealing with? How well are his coping mechanisms working? Does he have adequate social supports? Information about his symptoms in the absence of the context of his current life situation is almost meaningless. However, great danger lies in getting caught up in the details of Mr. Jones's experience. Many practitioners are reluctant to explore the psychosocial aspects of a patient's problem because when patients are encouraged to talk, they often consume great amounts of the practitioner's time without coming to any resolution. This leaves the practitioner behind schedule and battle weary with no satisfaction of having "treated" anything specific.

Sometimes we can intervene to reduce the stress, for example by asking family members to make certain adjustments, or by writing an excuse to relieve pressures at work. However, it may be more constructive to suggest ways to modify the perception of the stress or to teach the patient stress management techniques. The stress remains the same but the allostatic load becomes less. The perception of the stress changes and the patient reacts differently. *Objectively, nothing is changed, but subjectively everything is changed.*

A third-year medical student interviewing patients in a local physician's office told the following story.

A 46-year-old woman came into the office complaining of low back pain and bilateral leg pain. She had had this pain for three days and it was getting worse. She said that the pain was constant, progressive, "twelve on a scale from zero to ten", it radiated down both legs, prevented sleep and was not relieved by anything (she had tried Tylenol, Naprosyn, and Advil). Never in her life had she had this kind of experience. She was in so much pain that she could not eat. She had started to limp that morning. After this full description I asked, "What else is happening in your life?" Her answer, "I'm having troubles at work – the other women working there do not like me." I asked, "How do you feel about that?" She said, "It makes me sad, angry and terribly frustrated." When I asked, "What troubles you the most?" she answered, "The pain is so bad that I can't work, but I really need this job to survive. I am afraid that I am going to get fired." She paused, and then added, "They would really like to see me get fired." I asked, "How are you handling that?" Her reply was, "Not very well. I feel totally stressed out." I told her that it sounded like a tough situation to be in and that it must be very hard for her to deal with.

When she left the office, she was not limping anymore. It was almost as though figuring out what was really troubling her had had a powerful effect.

THE MEDICAL VISIT AS A STRESSFUL EVENT

For patients, there may be many sources of stress related to the office visit. First, the logistics of the visit including getting an appointment, taking time off from work, transportation, waiting time, forms to be filled out, and insurance hassles. Then the pain or anxiety related to the symptoms of illness or the presenting complaint. Another category concerns the *interpersonal elements* of the visit. Patients may feel stressed as they anticipate questions, judgments, scolding, praise, instructions and/or the diagnosis. Negative past experiences with physicians may arouse the fight or flight response and precipitate unpleasant bodily sensations.

Patients may feel anxious in anticipation of having to reveal personal information or parts of the body interpreting this as physical and emotional exposure. They anticipate demands to accept the authority of the practitioner, to follow instructions, to be a "good" patient. The patient may feel stressed in the dependent role, being out of control in this situation. The "White-Coat Hypertension Response" literature documents that approximately 40% of patients have systolic or diastolic blood pressure readings in the office setting that are at least 10 points higher than readings taken at home.[10,11]

Minimizing the Patient's Stress

A classic article in the *Journal of the American Medical Association* cited the effectiveness of empathic understanding in calming anxious patients.[12] Key phrases can be used to address a patient's response to a stressful situation, to make it overt and normalize it. As stated earlier, just recognizing a situation as a

26

problem changes it. By acknowledging, "It must be difficult for you to get here in the middle of your busy day," or, "You have had to wait a long time and must be quite impatient," the practitioner provides support and helps the patient to relax. An apology for making a patient wait goes a long way as well.

In the real world of every day practice, unfortunately, if practitioners address the issue of patient inconvenience at all, instead of focusing on the patient's experience and providing empathy, practitioners often explain why they were detained and cite emergencies or situations involving other patients with acute needs. This underscores the practitioner's importance, minimizes the patient's significance and increases the stress of the situation. These concepts will be discussed further in subsequent chapters.

Acceptance Is Key

When we acknowledge that the patient has a right to be annoyed or upset by having to wait, we have given support. One element of support is acceptance of a person's behavior. In giving support, we provide psychological relief. It is important to recognize and accept reactions rather than explain them. As Fritz Perls[13] has emphatically stated, it is the *what* and *how* that are important, not the *why*. Rather than trying to talk patients out of how they feel, or figuring out why they feel that way, we acknowledge those feelings and respond to them in a practical, therapeutic, time-effective way.

Many issues determine the patient's expectations in the doctor/patient relationship. These issues include patients' illness stories,[14,15] their requests,[16] and various explanatory models of illness growing out of the patient's cultural heritage.[17] Full discussion of these elements is beyond the scope of this book. However, whenever patients exhibit anxiety in the office, regardless of the source, it is most important *not* to say, "You have no reason to feel anxious!" If the patient actually had no reason to feel anxious, the patient would not feel that way. Instead, we recommend saying, "I can understand that you would feel anxious in this situation. Let's see what we can do to make you feel better."

WHY PATIENTS ADAPT DIFFERENTLY TO STRESS

When mental health is poor individuals are more likely to develop disease, and are much less tolerant of physical symptoms.[18,19] The correlation between illness and stressful life events is generally accepted. Holmes, Treuting, and Wolff, in 1951, first documented the effects of life situations and the accompanying emotional reactions on patients with hay fever.[20] Holmes and Rahe[21] standardized the schedule of recent life events that has been widely used in research. Still, many people under stress do not succumb to disease. They seem to resist diseases developed by others, and seem to prosper both physically and mentally, even under traumatic conditions. What makes them so different?

The "salutogenic" Model

The sociologist, Aaron Antonovsky,[22] studied the factors that seem to protect people from the consequences of stress, developing a "salutogenic" as opposed to "pathogenic" model. In explaining why some people stay healthy regardless of what happens to them, Antonovsky first specifies what he calls generalized resistance resources such as constitutionally good health, knowledge/intelligence, education, access to money, and a rational, flexible, and farsighted coping style. Given a sufficient amount of quality generalized resistance resources in childhood and adolescence, the individual will develop what Antonovsky calls a "sense of coherence." This characteristic seems to insulate a person from having negative health consequences, even from stressful events that cause disease in people who are more vulnerable. The sense of coherence is basically a stable psychological orientation allowing individuals to make sense out of different aspects of their lives, weaving their experience into a coherent whole. They are able to look at their lives and maintain a basic faith that, generally, "things will work out as well as can reasonably be expected," that everything happens for a reason, and consider that to be all right. A strong sense of coherence has been shown to predict good health in both men and women.[23] In clinical practice, this sense of coherence is an important concept that can be applied therapeutically, as will be discussed later.

Connection and Hardiness

To be able to connect aspects of our experience into a coherent whole is important as is connecting to other people. It is the loss of the sense of being connected that seems to be a critical factor in feeling and becoming vulnerable. Cassel[24] described this phenomenon, suggesting that the subjective interpretation, or personal experience, of an ill person induces a loss of connectedness. It is interesting to note that Kobasa's[25] original concept of hardiness specified qualities of commitment, challenge, control, and connection. Hardiness distinguishes people who do not succumb to illness under stress from those who do succumb. Hardy personalities find ways to make a meaningful commitment to the task, retain a sense of perceived control by focusing on their own behavior, redefine situations as a challenge, and connect with other people in supportive ways. Based on *hardiness* scores, Kobasa, Maddi, and Courington[26] were able to predict differences in illness response among executives stressed by similar life changes. It is the sensed loss of control that may make a person vulnerable, by compromising the immune system.

A Look at the Data

Now we wish to discuss several sets of research findings. First, we'll examine a prospective, longitudinal study that relates mental and physical health.[27,28] Next, we will discuss both theoretical and empirical data which indicate that every person has at least two levels of functioning. And finally, we will show how functioning under stress is related to the person's locus of control.[29]

A Longitudinal Study of Adaptation

In his book, *Adaptation to Life*,[27] George Vaillant described the details of the lives of a large number of subjects in the Grant Study of Adult Development, a comprehensive prospective study which followed 237 college men, who were healthy at the start of the study, for 55 years. Baseline data was collected through repeated physical examinations and by interviews and comprehensive questionnaires for the longitudinal monitoring of psychological, social, and occupational adjustments. All important life events were followed, as were the types of symptoms that the subjects developed under stress. This research clearly demonstrated the connection between healthy psychological and healthy physical functioning. Ultimately Vaillant concluded that there was little evidence to support the existence of specific mental diseases, only evidence of maladaptive reactions to stress.

Vaillant found that people change over time, generally "maturing" psychologically as they grow older. He also found that some people are healthier than others. Under favorable circumstances, mental health develops and is correlated with robust physical health. This also generally predisposes the person to success in the work environment. Both physical and mental health are dependent on successful adaptation. Poor physical health was followed by poor mental health. Conversely, poor mental health, i.e., poor adaptation to stressful life events, was a clear predictor of subsequent poor physical health. In a follow-up after 45 years of the study,[28] psychosocial factors gathered before age 50 were examined in relation to physical health, mental health and life satisfaction at age 65. Interestingly, the extent of tranquilizer use before age 50 (hardly the best response to managing stress) was the most powerful *negative* predictor of both physical and mental health. Paradoxically, a warm, supportive childhood environment made an important independent contribution to predicting *physical* health. In the most recent follow-up after 55 years of the study,[30] Vaillant found that a group of 64 men who had never used mood-altering drugs or consulted a psychiatrist before the age of 50 had significantly better health and lower mortality at age 70 than the rest of the group.

Successful Adaptation Defines Health

In a key finding, Vaillant reported that individual traumatic incidents did not generally have dramatic effects on the quality of people's lives. Rather, that people's lives, in general, seemed to have a relatively stable course.[27] The major finding of this study is that successfully adapting to problems, not the absence of stressors, determines healthy functioning and growth. Vaillant cited a range of adaptive mechanisms, which can also be labeled defense mechanisms. He proposed four lines of defenses: psychotic, immature, neurotic, and mature. We would like to discuss these concepts in somewhat greater detail.

Defense mechanisms such as delusional projection, denial, and distortion, that are part of the psychotic level, are normal for individuals under the age of five. These mechanisms are labeled "psychotic" because they dramatically alter what is generally perceived as reality. Immature mechanisms such as projection (taking unacceptable feelings and attributing them to others), hypochondriasis (focusing on subtle physical symptoms and assuming that serious undiagnosed disease is present), and acting out (turning feelings into generally unacceptable behavior) are common in healthy three- to 15-year-olds. The "neurotic" defenses outlined by Vaillant are the intellectualization (rationalization), repression (unconsciously keeping unacceptable feelings out of awareness), and reaction formation (countering bad impulses by doing the exact opposite), which are commonly seen in "healthy individuals ages three to 90, in neurotic disorders and in mastering acute adult stress."[31] Mature mechanisms such as altruism, humor, suppression (choosing not to think about something), anticipation, and sublimation (using the emotional energy in a productive way) are normal in healthy individuals from 12 to 90. Under stress, however, even healthy individuals may fall back on less mature mechanisms. When increased demands from the internal or external environments overcome the mature defense mechanisms, the individual temporarily retreats to more primitive defenses, regressing, or under severe conditions, decompensating (totally falling apart).

Extreme stress, and the price the body pays, now understood as allostatic load, is marked by individuals regressing from their characteristic coping mechanisms to less mature ones. These primitive coping mechanisms provide less successful adaptation further increasing the allostatic load and put the individual at risk for poorer mental and physical health. The most important finding according to Vaillant[27] is not that stress kills us, but that ingenious adaptation to stress, which he calls good mental health, facilitates our survival. Vaillant's work provides support for the themes that are central to this text:

1. mental and physical health are inextricably linked
2. individuals use different coping mechanisms under stress than when not under stress
3. in general, individuals have consistent coping patterns. They use specific patterns at a particular level of maturity under normal circumstances and less functional ones under stress
4. it is critical to support people under stress in order to help them return to more adaptive defenses and functioning.

A Holistic Theory of Neurosis

Vaillant comes from a psychoanalytic school of psychiatry. We shall now look at a psychiatrist with a very different orientation, who provides interesting theoretical support for the conclusions of the Grant study.

Andras Angyal's work is not well known in the medical community. Angyal[32] was a successful analyst who proposed a theory and treatment of neurosis that he labeled a holistic method. His theory is useful because it provides a plausible explanation for the uncomfortable phenomena that people experience when they are under overwhelming stress. Angyal also provides direction for producing relief.

Angyal's theory of human nature and personality posits that two systems, one healthy and one neurotic, vie for dominance in our personality. All persons have a need to feel competent, or as Angyal puts it, there is a drive for autonomy. There is also a companion need to belong, which Angyal calls the need for homonomy, essentially a feeling of connectedness. The healthy system develops through the experience of having one's basic needs met, that is, both feeling personally competent and also feeling accepted by the significant others in one's life. The healthy system is based on both feeling loved (connected) and effective as an autonomous person (competent). The world of the healthy personality is a reasonably safe and loving place. Conversely, the neurotic system builds on experiences of feeling incompetent, rejected or resentful. It registers only needs that have been unfulfilled. Angyal suggests that since no life, however unfortunate, consists solely of trauma, the basic data processed by the two systems is identical. Angyal says that we actually live in two worlds. Both are complete systems and they vie for dominance. We never live in the world proper, but create our map of the world,[33] a map that is not the same as the territory.[34] Moreover, Angyal now tells us that we actually have two different maps, which we use under different circumstances.

We either relate to the world with reasonably positive expectations using our healthy map, or with unreasonable fear and discomfort using our neurotic map. When the neurotic system is engaged, the world seems hostile, threatening, and withholding, and our primary aim is to protect ourselves and escape danger. The world feels huge and menacing while we feel small and inadequate. This belief system prevents us from feeling safe or optimistic. Danger exists everywhere. Until our healthy self has been re-engaged, we cannot feel hope or problem solve confidently.

Support helps to restore people's sense of trust in the world that is represented by the healthy personality system. Therapeutic interventions that cause patients to feel competent and connected will re-engage their healthy systems.

Research from Experimental Psychology

Although shaped in different language, physiological experimental psychology has demonstrated specific responses in subjects under stress. As people become over aroused (tense and over stimulated), they filter out parts of current experience: coping mechanisms become more primitive in several ways including reversion to more dominant, first learned behaviors. When recently learned behavior is not available, those responses that might be most appropriate to the situation are temporarily blocked and cannot be utilized. Novel stimuli are not recognized. Under highly aroused conditions, people revert to "over-learned" responses. This means they automatically use behavior that has been repeated so often that it requires no conscious thought.[35] When levels of arousal return to a comfortable level, problem solving becomes effective again. Recently learned material is back in the behavioral repertoire, increasing available options. Mental health is restored.

31

Therapeutic Implication

The connecting thread between these viewpoints confirms our personal clinical experience that facing unmanageable stressors puts people on "tilt." For many people there are degrees of diminishing functioning under stress, perhaps even a peak of efficiency before the decline sets in, but everyone has their threshold that precipitates behavior characteristic of overstressed functioning. Having passed this threshold, people click in their neurotic map of the world, acting as though this were the only reality they knew. For the clinician, the primary therapeutic task is to provide support in order to restore people's equilibrium and reestablish them in their healthier orientation. This is often not difficult. Weick has pointed out that simply labeling a problem as minor rather than serious lowers people's arousal level. He suggested that this is particularly beneficial when "people don't know what to do or are unable to do it."[36]

Internal or External Locus of Control

People's health-related behavior is strongly influenced by their locus of control, an important construct that few practitioners apply with awareness. Individuals with an internal locus of control[37] cope best when they have the resources (information, power, time) to handle a situation, whereas individuals with an external locus of control, feel safe when a trusted authority figure has taken charge and told them what to do, or when family or community resources have been recruited for their support.[38] Because locus of control influences people's reactions to stressful circumstances, the implications for medical practice and for dealing with patients and others under stress are obvious.

Keeping these concepts in mind – the relationship between psychological and physical well-being, the regression to primitive functioning whenever defenses are overwhelmed, and security based on internal or external locus of control – will enable you to make effective interventions, at critical times, with little investment of time, energy, or effort.

APPLICATION TO ILLNESS BEHAVIOR

The effects of acute illness constitute a high degree of stress. People's behavior when they are sick can be better understood by looking at the process of normal maturity. Chris Argyris, writing from the point of view of organizational psychology, specified five dimensions of individual development.[39] As people mature, they move along a continuum from being passive to being active; from dependence to independence; from needing immediate gratification to being able to delay gratification for long periods; from concrete thinking to abstract thinking; and from having few abilities to having many abilities. At any given time, each person functions at a specific level on each of these dimensions. The more highly developed or mature the individual, the higher the level of functioning along each axis that can be expected. In circumstances of acute stress, people will temporarily regress along each of the five dimensions, though not necessarily to the same extent. Vaillant's findings confirmed this phenomenon.[27]

Acute illness may precipitate an acute regression of functioning. People who are ill become more passive, more dependent, want their demands met instantly, become more concrete in their thinking and have fewer abilities to help themselves. This can try the patience of the caregiver, but can be better handled if it is anticipated and perceived to be transitory. In chronic illness, unfortunately, the regression often becomes permanent. Practitioners aware of this dynamic can prevent further stress by helping caregivers to set realistic expectations for the patient and the course of the illness, and encouraging the return to premorbid levels of functioning.

Results of Being Overwhelmed

The subjective feeling of being overwhelmed contributes to the objective inability of individuals to function at optimum levels. The resulting perception of inadequacy lowers the individual's sense of self-esteem. These feelings can be transient; lasting only several seconds, or may constitute the general phenomenological experience of the individual. Often negative experiences of the self are specific to particular symbolically threatening situations. At other times, they may be precipitated and maintained by traumatic life events or by an accumulation of daily hassles. No particular situation or event is considered to be inherently stressful, rather it is the individual's interpretation of the situation as threatening or harmful that defines it as a stressor.[40] William James first suggested that emotions and their effects on our bodies are objective phenomena that are determined through the subjective experience:

> Our natural way of thinking about these . . . emotions is that the mental perception of some fact excites the mental affection called the emotion, and that this latter state of mind gives rise to the bodily expression. My theory on the contrary, is that the bodily changes follow directly on the perception of the exciting fact, and that our feeling of the same changes as they occur IS the emotion. Common sense says we lose our fortune, are sorry and weep; we meet a bear, are frightened, and run; we are insulted by a rival, are angry, and strike. The hypothesis here to be defended says that this order of sequence is incorrect, that the one mental state is not immediately induced by the other, that the bodily manifestations must first be interposed between, and that the more rational statement is that we feel sorry because we cry, angry because we strike, or tremble because we are sorry, angry, or fearful, as the case may be. Without the bodily states following on the perception, the latter would be purely cognitive in form, pale, colorless, destitute of emotional warmth. We might then see the bear, and judge it best to run, receive the insult and deem it right to strike, but we should not actually feel afraid or angry.[41]

When we feel basically in control of our responses to the events happening in our lives, appropriately able to flee, fight, or flow, we function at an effective level. As long as the demands of the external environment (other people) and internal environment (expectations for the self) are experienced as manageable, we will continue to function at our customary level. Once the tolerance for comfortable adaptation has been exceeded, however, we begin to use a different coping style. At the extreme, Martin Seligman has shown that once people are convinced that events are completely beyond their control and that their behavior will in no way affect the outcome of a particular situation, they behave in a stereotypical manner that he has labeled "learned helplessness."[42] Learned helplessness is an emotional sequence that involves going through a fear-protest stage to a helpless-depressed stage. The more out of control the person feels, the more primitive are the defenses called into play. Although this response appears to be ineffective, it is a person's best effort to survive when in an overwhelmed state.

Each of us can usually identify when we are feeling overwhelmed by observing our behavior. We go on *tilt*, and are temporarily unable to do anything about it. Sometimes our awareness can help us engage strategies to restore our equilibrium. In many cases, however, our perception of our behavior, and our inability to control or modify it, exacerbate the feelings of being overwhelmed. When we lose faith in our power to manage at all, we fall into our dependent mode, and look to be taken care of. When there is no one to do this, or when we do not trust the person who is in charge, we become despondent and helpless.

At first, patients are simply aware of symptoms such as muscle tension, which may be experienced as back, neck or head pain. Patients may become aware of a rapid pulse, abdominal pain, breathing difficulties, blurred vision, a full bladder, diarrhea, sweating, tight throat or they may have trouble swallowing. Other less noticeable bodily reactions triggered by the sympathetic nervous system-mediated stress-response may result in elevated blood pressure, elevated lipid levels, change in blood sugar, suppression of the immune system, and ultimately the compromise of various organ systems. The bi-directional communication between the brain and the immune system is now well established.[43,44]

THE CRISIS INTERVENTION MODEL

A crisis may be thought of as an environmentally produced situation to which the individual must respond, such as a disaster, an accident, the loss of a job or the death of a loved one. There are also normal developmental crises (also called transition points) in the life cycle. A crisis may be thought of most simply as the time of greatest change or potential change, often creating emotional upset, increased tension, unpleasant affect, coping mechanisms breakdown and disorganized functioning. A situation is experienced as a crisis when an individual perceives an event as threatening to the self in some significant way. It is a time of acute stress. People present to a primary care provider in crisis, but generally come in complaining of organic problems. First one must identify the precipitant and then seize the opportunity to be therapeutic. Crisis is a time when certain decisions must be made because the previous *status quo* no longer exists. These decisions are important since they will affect subsequent options available. However, crisis is also a time when because of the emotional overlay, the individual is least capable of thinking clearly or problem solving effectively.

Gerald Caplan,[45] explaining the effectiveness of crisis intervention, suggests that each person generally functions within a specific range of effectiveness and personal satisfaction. We have seen this empirically demonstrated by Vaillant.[27,28] There is a continuum of functioning, from people who are generally very ineffective to those who are well-adjusted and adapted and who enjoy living. In general, people are quite static in their level of functioning, regularly fluctuating within a given range as they experience manageable life stress. As stated previously, in a crisis there is an overwhelming amount of emotional distress and the individual is unable to process information objectively or solve problems effectively. Since a crisis is defined as the time of greatest change, regardless of the nature or degree of adaptation required, crisis by definition is time-limited. Some resolution will occur within a time-span of four to six weeks. The distressed individual is generally eager to receive help, having temporarily moved down on the dependency scale. This affords the clinician an opportunity to intervene effectively at a time when the individual is open and highly suggestible.

The Goal of Crisis Intervention

Crisis intervention aims to achieve very specific and limited outcomes. There are four general objectives. The first is to prevent dire consequences. In a crisis, the individual is forced to deal with new situations just at a time when the ability to solve problems is compromised. The intervening person can suggest that no decision be made that is not absolutely crucial, and that those issues that must be resolved are talked through carefully with a disinterested person.

The second objective is to return the individual to the premorbid level of functioning. As we have discussed previously, providing support that makes the person feel competent and connected will help to achieve this outcome. Expanding the behavioral repertoire and enhancing self-esteem are the two other objectives of crisis intervention. Weathering the crisis, finding new ways to manage problems and negotiate personal relationships not only expands the behavioral repertoire, but also creates a positive change in self-esteem and the sense of self-efficacy.

Symptom relief along with empathy for the subjective experiences of distress is also important. Additionally, the clinician can provide information and explanations, explore options, or simply point out that options exist and prescribe "tincture of time." Most of all, the practitioner can encourage new behavior to help the patient manage the crisis and attain a better level of functioning when psychological and physical equilibrium are restored.

Expected Outcomes

If the resolution of the crisis is favorable, the individual can be expected to function at a higher level of adjustment. New coping skills are learned and confidence in self and others is enhanced. Conversely, if there is no help available, or if the individual is unable to solve the problem successfully, with or without help, because by definition crises are time limited, the situation will still be resolved, but at the cost of a subsequent lower level of functioning. People will move down the scale in all five of Argyris's[37] dimensions.

It is important to remember that during a time of crisis a person experiences increased dependency needs, wishes to be helped, and signals this to the environment. One of the most efficient ways of signaling for help in our society is to develop an illness, either an acute illness or the exacerbation of a chronic condition. The primary care visit is a cry for help, and for symptom relief. It affords the aware practitioner a unique opportunity to invest a few minutes making a therapeutic intervention that has the potential to provide both short-term and long-term benefits for the patient.

APPLICATION TO THE OFFICE SETTING

Some patients at first seem reluctant to discuss their psychological condition when they seek medical treatment. The following example is quite typical of our practice.

Mrs. Z is a 53-year-old schoolteacher who has come to the office for the second time. Her presenting complaint is a sinus problem; she reports having had congestion and severe recurrent headaches for the past three days. Mrs. Z has a history of chronic sinusitis, but this time she says the symptoms have persisted for a longer time than usual. Mrs. Z is a well-dressed, reserved white female who appears somewhat anxious to get out of the office. When she is asked about her current life situation, she reluctantly admits that she is working two jobs, is separated from her husband, but states that everything is under control. She refuses to give any details of her current situation and when asked how she feels about her separation she denies that she has any problems, and says that she doesn't want to talk about it. Physical exam is normal. The practitioner then explains to her that sometimes stress and emotional problems have a way of lowering the body's resistance and making physical symptoms persist longer or be more difficult to treat. If these problems are not recognized and dealt with, physical health is compromised. The practitioner just presents this explanation to help the patient make sense out of both her current situation and her reaction to it. Deciding to give the patient a few minutes to think about it, he then leaves the room to get a prescription. When he returns, he notices that the patient is looking much more relaxed. She says, "Doctor, I really didn't mind you asking me questions about my separation and so forth. It was good that you did.

I really have to start dealing with all that stuff." The doctor then schedules her for an appointment the following week, primarily to talk about her psychosocial situation. She leaves feeling much better.

We have tried to show that the practitioner usually sees patients at a time when they are feeling vulnerable. Interventions at this time are very effective, both in restoring the patient's equilibrium and promoting constructive change. The therapeutic goal is always to make the patient feel both competent and connected. Specific techniques and detailed rationale will be discussed in subsequent chapters. The practitioner is in a unique position to help the patient at an opportune time and is equipped with a variety of valuable skills, as will be discussed in the next chapter.

SUMMARY

The stress response is a biologically programmed mobilization for adaptive action in response to changes in the external or internal environments. The cost of coping with chronic or cumulative stress differs among individuals and the resulting price paid by the body has been defined as "allostatic load." The visit to the practitioner is often triggered by distress felt in response to situational factors. Patients also experience stress in regard to the office visit and their interaction with the practitioner. This can be reduced by specific strategies.

In general, there is a relationship between illness and adaptation to life events. Good mental health potentiates physical well-being. Some people are characteristically healthier than others. Drawing from a variety of sources, we present two central concepts: first, that individuals generally function at a specific level of adaptation and second, that individuals under severe stress, including physical illness, temporarily regress to lower levels of functioning. People with internal locus of control primarily need to feel competent and in control while people with external locus of control primarily need to feel connected to a trusted caretaker.

Based on previous experiences and in reaction to life circumstances, people either relate to the world with positive expectations using their healthy map, or with fear and discomfort, using their neurotic map. When individuals are in a state of being overwhelmed, they are unable to function at optimum levels. They go on *tilt* and engage their neurotic map of the world. Until their healthy self is reengaged, they cannot feel hope or confidence. Social support, which provides information regarding an individual's basic acceptability and competence, is crucial at this time.

The crisis intervention model is useful in specifying the time-limited nature of acute stress. Crises generally resolve within four to six weeks. By providing support, crisis intervention aims to prevent dire consequences, return the individual to a premorbid level of functioning, to enhance self-esteem, and expand subsequent coping abilities. If practitioners understand these mechanisms and routinely provide supportive interventions, the results will be therapeutic for patients and rewarding for the practitioner.

The role of the supportive person is to restore the sense of trust in the world that is represented by the healthy personality system. When the actions of the practitioner make the patient feel competent and connected, the healthy system will be reengaged.

References

1. APA Press Release: Stress a major health problem in the U.S. Available at: www. apa.org/releases/stressproblem.html (accessed 24 October 2007).
2. Selye H. *The Stress of Life.* New York: McGraw-Hill; 1957.
3. McEwen BS. The neurobiology of stress: from serendipity to clinical relevance. *Brain Res.* 2000; **886**(1-2): 172–89.
4. Griffen KW, Friend R, Kaell AT, *et al.* Distress and disease status among patients with rheumatoid arthritis: roles of coping styles and perceived responses from support providers. *Ann Behav Med.* 2001; **23**: 133–8.
5. Kroenke CH, Kubzansky LD, Schernhammer ES, *et al.* Social networks, social support, and survival after breast cancer diagnosis. *J Clin Oncol.* 2006; **24**(7): 1105–11.
6. Cohen S, Doyle WJ, Skoner, DP, *et al.* Social ties and susceptibility to the common cold. *JAMA.* 1997; **277**(24): 1940–4.
7. Tennant C. Life stress, social support and coronary heart disease. *Aust N Z J Psychiatry.* 1999; **33**: 636–41.
8. Price MA, Tennant CC, Butow PN, *et al.* The role of psychosocial factors in the development of breast carcinoma: Part II. Life event stressors, social support, defense style, and emotional control and their interactions. *Cancer.* 2001; **91**: 686–97.
9. Feldman PJ, Dunkel-Schetter C, Sandman, CA *et al.* Maternal social support predicts birth weight and fetal growth in human pregnancy. *Psychosom Med.* 2000; **62**: 715–25.
10. Lerman CE, Brody DS, Hui T, *et al.* The white-coat hypertension response: prevalence and predictors. *J Gen Intern Med.* 1989; **4**: 226–31.
11. MacDonald MB, Laing GP, Wilson MP, *et al.* Prevalence and predictors of the white coat response in patients with treated hypertension. *Can Med Ass J.* 1999; **161**(3): 265–9.
12. Bellet PS, Maloney MJ. The importance of empathy as an interviewing skill in medicine. *JAMA.* 1991; **266**:1831–2.
13. Perls FS. *Gestalt Therapy Verbatim.* Moab, Utah: Real People Press; 1969.
14. Brody H. *Stories of Sickness.* New Haven, Conn.: Yale University Press; 1987.
15. Kleinman A. *The Illness Narratives.* New York: Basic Books; 1988.
16. Lazare A, Eisenthal S. A negotiated approach to the clinical encounter I: Attending the patient's perspective. In: Lazare A, (ed.) *Outpatient Psychiatry.* Baltimore: Williams & Wilkins; 1979. pp. 157–71.
17. Mechanic D. Response factors in illness: the studies of illness behavior. In: Jaco G, (ed.) *Patients, Practitioners, Illness: a source book in behavioral science and health.* New York: The Free Press; 1979.
18. Vaillant GE. Natural history of male psychologic health: effects of mental health on physical health. *N Eng J Med.* 1979; **301**: 1249–54.

19. Vaillant GE, Gerber PD. Natural history of male psychological health XIV: relationship of mood disorder vulnerability to physical health. *Am J Psychiatry.* 1998; **155**: 184–91.

20. Holmes TH, Treuting T, Wolff HG. Life situations, emotions and nasal disease: evidence on summative effects exhibited in patients with "hay fever." *Psychosom Med.* 1951; **13**: 71–82.

21. Holmes TH, Rahe RH. The social readjustment rating scale. *Psychosom Med.* 1967; **11**: 213–18.

22. Antonovsky A. *Unraveling the Mystery of Health: how people manage stress and stay well.* San Francisco: Jossey-Bass Publishers; 1987.

23. Suominen S, Helenius H, Blomberg H, *et al.* Sense of coherence as a predictor of subjective state of health: results of 4 years of follow-up of adults. *J Psychosom Res.* 2001; **50**: 77–86.

24. Cassel J. The contribution of the social environment to host resistance. *Am J Epidem.* 1976; **104**: 107–23.

25. Kobasa SC. Stressful life events, personality, and health: an inquiry into hardiness. *J Pers Soc Psych.* 1979; **37**: 1–11.

26. Kobasa SC, Maddi SR, Courington S. Personality and constitution as mediators in the stress-illness relationship. *J Health Soc Behavior.* 1981; **22**: 368–78.

27. Vaillant GE. *Adaptation to Life.* Boston: Little, Brown & Co.; 1977.

28. Vaillant GE, Vaillant CO. Natural history of male psychological health XII: a 45-year study of predictors of successful aging at age 65. *Am J Psychiatry.* 1990; **147**: 31–7.

29. Rotter JB. Generalized expectancies for internal versus external control of reinforcement. *Psychol Monogr.* 1966; **80**(1): 1–28.

30. Vaillant GE. *Aging Well: surprising guideposts to a happier life from the landmark Harvard Study of Adult Development.* Boston: Little, Brown; 2003.

31. Vaillant GE. *Adaptation to Life,* op. cit. p. 384.

32. Angyal A. *Neurosis and Treatment: a holistic theory.* New York: John Wiley & Sons, Inc.; 1965.

33. Korzybski A. *Science & Sanity.* 4th ed. Lakeville, Connecticut: The International Non-Aristotelian Library Publishing Company; 1958.

34. Bateson G. *Mind and Nature: a necessary unity.* New York: E. P. Dutton; 1979.

35. Staw BM, Sandelands LE, Dutton JE. Threat-rigidity effects in organizational behavior: a multilevel analysis. *Admin Sci Quart.* 1981; **26**: 501–24.

36. Weick KE. Small wins: redefining the scale of social problems. *Am Psychol.* 1984; **39**: 41.

37. Wallston BS, Wallston KA, Kaplan GD, *et al.* Development and validation of the health locus of control (HCL) scale. *J Consult Clin Psychol.* 1976; **44**: 580–5.

38. Janz NK, Becker MH. The health belief model: a decade later. *Health Educ Q.* 1984; **11**: 1–47.

39. Argyris C. *Intervention Theory and Method: a behavioral science view.* Reading, MA: Addison-Wesley; 1970.

40. Zakowski SG, Hall MK, Klein LC, *et al.* Appraised control, coping and stress in a community sample: a test of the goodness-of-fit-hypothesis. *Ann Behav Med.* 2001; **23**(3): 158–65.

41. James W. *The Principles of Psychology, Vol. 2.* New York: Holt; 1913 (no. 1). pp. 449–50.

42. Seligman MEP *Helplessness: on depression, development, and death.* San Francisco: Freeman; 1975.

43. Maier SF, Watkins LR. Cytokines for psychologists: implications of bidirectional immune-to-brain communication for understanding behavior, mood and cognition. *Psychol Rev.* 1998; **105**(1): 83–107.

44. Baratta MV, Christianson JP, Gomez DM, *et al.* Controllable versus uncontrollable stressors bi-directionally modulate conditioned but not innate fear. *Neuroscience* 2007; **146**(4): 1495–503.

45. Caplan G. *Principles of Preventive Psychiatry.* New York: Basic Books; 1964.

CHAPTER 3

Cognitive Behavioral Therapy and Other Practical Therapeutic Interventions

In this age of evidence-based medicine, cognitive behavioral therapy has become the most highly recommended form of non-pharmacological treatment of anxiety, depressive and other mental health disorders.[1] This chapter will clarify the power of some of these techniques as well as specifying what the term "practical therapeutic interventions" implies. Our goal is to prepare you to use your interview with the patient to precipitate positive change in patients' views of themselves, their situations and their options. This is the essence of "psychotherapy."

In our many workshops based on *The Fifteen Minute Hour*, participants tell us that they feel uncomfortable with the word "psychotherapy." They prefer to use the word "counseling." We make the distinction that counseling refers to giving patients suggestions or advice, whereas psychotherapy, or therapeutic intervention, implies deliberately using psychological techniques to attempt to modify how patients view themselves, their world, and their options in that world. We want practitioners to be aware that words when used deliberately have the same potential as procedures to markedly affect patients' views of their current reality.

J.D. Frank, in the revised edition of *Persuasion and Healing*, defines psychotherapy as influence characterized by three elements: first, a trained, socially sanctioned healer, whose healing powers are accepted by the sufferer; second, a sufferer who seeks relief from the sanctioned healer; and finally a circumscribed series of contacts between the healer and the sufferer. He suggests that the efficacy of psychotherapy is based on the shared belief of the participants that these methods will work.[2] It is our contention that contacts between patients and primary care practitioners whose intention is to provide psychological support fulfill these criteria.

Since psychological factors both predispose the patient to illness and affect recovery from illness, interventions designed to decrease psychological pain or dysfunction play a critical role in good medical treatment. Psychotherapy can be understood as a process that uses a variety of verbal and nonverbal messages to empower patients. It enables patients to increase their trust in themselves and others, validates their feelings, enhances their sense of self-esteem, diminishes their feelings of isolation or depression, and helps them develop a sense of purpose, put it into action, and to manage their stress. We will identify specific, practical techniques, including Cognitive Behavioral Therapy (CBT) that can effectively be incorporated into the brief primary care office visit.

To reiterate, psychotherapy consists of the things we say – and the processes of how we say them – that make the patient feel better. Our interaction with the patient, the therapeutic talk, has an ameliorating effect on the patient's distress. Different schools of psychiatry and psychology will claim that training and supervision in their particular method of psychotherapy are the critical factors in precipitating the change in self-image, world view, emotional response, or overt behavior that is associated with a successful outcome in psychotherapy. We maintain that certain universal influences can be used therapeutically and that understanding these dynamics and applying them intentionally potentiates healing.

HUMAN BEINGS TELL STORIES

Every one of us makes assumptions about the nature of the world based on our personal experiences starting in early childhood. Much of this process is out of the level of awareness. Then, as psychotherapist John Welwood puts it:

> We perpetuate these conditioned ways of perceiving the world through repetitive stories we tell ourselves about "the way things are." These kinds of stories are mental fabrications, judgments or interpretations that put what is happening into a familiar framework. Usually we do not recognize these stories as our own invention; instead, we believe that they represent reality.[3]

The more neurotic people are, the more distorted their world view and the more limited their stories. Patients never question these stories about who they are and what they are or are not capable of doing, yet these stories place limits on subsequent experiences and behaviors. Psychotherapy in general and CBT in particular focus on challenging these stories.

Psychotherapy Means Editing the Story

Psychotherapy helps to change the stories that patients tell themselves. We like to define psychotherapy as what we do to "fix" patients' maps of the world so that they can figure out the best way to go in order to get what they want. Research has

42

overwhelmingly demonstrated the effectiveness of psychotherapy over placebo or no-treatment approaches, but little evidence demonstrates the superiority of one type of therapy over another.[4] Certain approaches, however, are more practical and lend themselves more effectively for use in primary care.

Our major concern is to describe and modify those therapeutic processes that work, regardless of the "brand name." The most effective techniques are generic. Our mission is to try to clarify what works, how to do it, and what might be accomplished, especially in the short run. So, how exactly might we define our goals?

Therapeutic Goals

Most simply put, the goal of therapeutic interventions is to make patients feel better, to lower their levels of distress, and combat their feelings of being overwhelmed. As pointed out in Chapter 2, when patients feel overwhelmed by the circumstances of their lives or their reaction to those circumstances, they develop a wide range of somatic and psychological symptoms. The most common symptoms from which patients suffer are anxiety and depression, which often occur simultaneously and may be accompanied by other somatic manifestations.[5] These symptoms develop because of patients' interpretations of their situation (their stories about the situation), not because of the situation itself. However, regardless of etiology, the experience of the symptoms further compromises patients' coping ability.

Patients Go on "tilt"

When patients' coping ability becomes overextended, they cease functioning effectively, a condition we label as *tilt*. The goal of psychotherapeutic intervention is to make the patient feel better and go off *tilt*. Feeling better in this connotation relates to the emotional or mental state of the patient. It means return to normal or base line functioning.

Specifically, we want to enhance patients' perceived personal power to deal with the circumstances of their lives. The sense of control has been shown to be the key factor in maintaining physical and mental health.[6] When people perceive themselves to be in control, whether they are or not, they function better. Perceived control has been shown to have a direct effect on autonomic reactivity and immune responses.[7] Perceived control enables a person to function better in response to demands from both the internal and external environments. At the least, it improves coping, which helps to restore the person's equilibrium, resulting in greater feelings of competence and belonging. Basically, our therapeutic goal is to help patients regain their sense of competence, so that they feel empowered to affect the course of their lives.

WHY IT IS IMPORTANT TO HAVE PATIENTS BACK IN CONTROL

Once the patient's psychological state improves, that patient not only will be able to function better in the realms of interpersonal relations and job performance, but also will be more effective in mobilizing the body's defenses in response to existent or potential disease.[8] We also know that a patient with an enhanced sense of well-being will sleep better, have a healthier appetite, and maintain a more reasonable flow of energy. In contrast to the vicious cycle of demoralization, depression, and compromised immune response leading to disease and further demoralization, the body's healthy defenses will be engaged, leading to a strengthened sense of personal competence and an improved ability to resist disease.

Often the psychotherapeutic intervention will cause patients to make positive changes in their assumptive world view, meaning that it will allow them to edit their stories and add positive chapters. This altered belief system then precipitates new ways of thinking and behaving that result in more satisfactory experiences, providing a natural reinforcement mechanism and instigating a benevolent circle.[9]

A physician in his third year of family practice training described the following case:

> The patient is a 62-year-old white male whom I had been seeing routinely for blood pressure checks. He has a history of hypertension and peptic ulcer disease. He is a rather stoic person who generally keeps his feelings to himself, and, as I found out, "somatizes" and develops symptoms. After seeing him several times for vague and persistent abdominal discomfort, I persisted in knowing what was going on in his life. He mentioned problems at work and at home and then unexpectedly added that the combination had made him impotent. When I asked him how that made him feel, he at first denied that it had any effect but then complained of headaches. Questioned about what troubled him the most, the patient said it was his impotence because he could not satisfy his wife, even with her reassurance that "it doesn't bother her." I then asked how he was handling this stress. He replied that he gets up and "walks it off." After assuring the patient that this must be very difficult, I taught him some progressive relaxation techniques to help manage his stress and after tapering all medications that could contribute to his impotence referred him to a urologist. The interesting thing is that in all subsequent visits he expects to be questioned about his stressors and considers it part of his treatment. Unfortunately, at present he is still impotent. Although there are no medical contraindications, he has repeatedly declined a prescription for sildenafil (Viagra), but there are no more complaints of abdominal pain or headaches.

Supportive Therapy

Traditionally, a broad distinction has been made between supportive psychotherapy and explorative psychotherapy. Before we discuss the generic elements of all psychotherapies, we would like to explain the differences between supportive and exploratory therapies. Supportive therapy is designed to restore premorbid or optimal functioning (making the patient feel competent and connected), whereas explorative therapy is concerned with uncovering personality patterns to understand the etiology of disorders (why the patient does not feel competent and connected). Techniques promoted by proponents of supportive therapy include abreaction (catharsis: giving patients a chance to talk about the problem), dependency (being there for the patient), exploration of symptomatology, encouragement of more productive behavior, and resolution through clarification. Basically, to be effective, all therapeutic interventions must be supportive, with the goal of helping patients to feel competent and connected.

Explorative Therapy

In explorative therapy the patient's behavior and feelings are examined from a historical perspective to help the patient develop insight. We cannot stress too strongly that insight or understanding by itself has no practical benefit because it does not necessarily change a patient's behavior. Watzlawick and his colleagues[10] in their book *Change: Principles of Problem Formation and Problem Resolution* make the following point:

> Everyday experience, not just clinical practice, shows that there can be change without insight. In fact, very few behavioral or social changes are accompanied, let alone preceded, by insight into the vicissitudes of their genesis. It may, for instance, be that the insomniac's difficulty has its roots in the past: his tired, nervous mother may habitually have yelled at him to sleep and to stop bothering her. But while this kind of discovery may provide a plausible and at times even very sophisticated explanation of a problem, it usually contributes nothing towards its solution. (p. 86.)

In a brilliant footnote these authors argue as follows:

> Such empirical findings . . . (must be) thought through to their logical conclusions. There are two possibilities: (1) The causal significance of the past is only a fascinating but inaccurate myth. In this case, the only question is the pragmatic one: How can desirable change of present behavior be most efficiently produced? (2) There is a causal relationship between the past and present behavior. But since past events are obviously unchangeable, either we are forced to abandon all hope that change is possible, or we must assume that – at least in

some significant respects – the past has influence over the present only by way of a person's present interpretation of past experience. If so, then the significance of the past becomes a matter not of "truth" and "reality," but of looking at it here and now in one way rather than another. Consequently, there is no compelling reason to assign to the past primacy or causality in relation to the present, and this means that the reinterpretation of the past is simply one of many ways of possibly influencing present behavior. In this case, then, we are back at the only meaningful question, i.e., the pragmatic one: How can desirable change of present behavior be produced most efficiently? (p. 86.)

So, contrary to conventional wisdom, the reason why people are behaving in a particular manner is irrelevant. If the behavior is destructive, it is important to help them to change it. (In some cases, very intellectual types may feel that they must understand why before they can bring themselves to change – but in the final analysis it is their decision to make a change that is effective, not understanding why they behaved the way they did in the first place.) The beauty of CBT is that the focus is on the story or how we think about a situation, and when that thinking changes, our reaction to the situation changes.

FIVE COMMON ELEMENTS IN EFFECTIVE PSYCHOTHERAPY
The field of the psychotherapies includes a wide variety of modalities and orientations. There is long-term, short-term, individual, group, couple, and family therapy. In any of these modalities, the orientation can be behavioral, interpersonal, psychoanalytical, gestalt, dynamic, cognitive, existential, narrative, schema-focused, rational emotive, or eclectic, to mention only a few. Regardless of theoretical orientation, certain basic principles and strategies are associated with the therapeutic change process.[11]

The Expectation of Receiving Help
Common to all psychotherapeutic modalities is the initially induced expectation that the therapy will be helpful. Jerome Frank[12] repeatedly pointed out that patients seek therapy because they are feeling helpless, hopeless, and demoralized. He specifically defined the demoralization commonly experienced by patients as "a state of subjective incapacity plus distress. The patient suffers from a sense of failure, loss of self-esteem, feelings of hopelessness or helplessness, and feelings of alienation or isolation. These are often accompanied by a sense of mental confusion, which the patient may express as a fear of insanity." The expectation that help is imminent helps to lift the patient from the depths of demoralization.

The Therapeutic Relationship

The second general principle associated with all psychotherapeutic modalities is the client's or patient's participation in a therapeutic relationship. This relationship exists for the sole purpose of fostering the well-being of the patient. A contract (or understanding) is made in which the clinician agrees to engage with the patient in a manner that fosters the expression of feelings and concerns in an accepting atmosphere. This contract for caring and concern is the core of therapy. The nature of the relationship determines the efficacy of the healing process. Regardless of theoretical orientation, from psychoanalytical to behavioral, it is the connection – the special relationship with the practitioner who communicates caring, understanding and respect for the patient, takes the patient seriously, and is devoted to the patient's welfare – that is the generic healing component.

Obtaining an External Perspective

The third factor found in all psychotherapies is giving patients the opportunity to obtain an external or objective perspective on their problems. By bringing their perceptions of their situation to a person not directly involved, patients are exposed to alternative interpretations, are made aware of potential options, and learn something about how other people might react to a similar situation. The external perspective affords patients the opportunity to check their possibly inaccurate perceptions of reality, the stories they are telling themselves about what is going on in their life. If the listener does not get upset when hearing about the "outrageous" situation the patient describes, the patient may conclude that there might be a reasonable way to react. Perhaps there is some hope after all.

Encouraging Corrective Experiences

All psychotherapeutic modalities encourage corrective experiences. It has been said that insanity consists of doing the same thing over and over again and expecting a different outcome. The definition of the corrective experience may vary according to the theoretical orientation of the practitioner. However, until learning is put into practice and changes how patients relate to themselves, their world, and the significant others in their lives, no healing occurs. The practitioner's role is to act as a consultant and cheerleader, encouraging patients to think and behave in new ways, and to define and achieve their goals. This is the essence of a corrective experience. Patients are coached to react to situations in less destructive ways. The benefits of this improved behavior include an enhanced sense of well-being and greater satisfaction from their interactions with others. These results then promote further gains.

Providing the Opportunity to Test Reality Repeatedly

The last principle common to all psychotherapies is the opportunity to test reality repeatedly. Patients' judgments of others, including others' intentions, are often quite inaccurate. These judgments are part of the story that the patients constantly repeat to themselves. An objective listener can confirm the reasonableness of the patients' reactions, challenge the accuracy of patients' conclusions, and/or suggest alternate interpretations. By examining their possibly faulty assumptions, the essence of CBT, patients are able to get a more accurate view of personal patterns of behavior, strengths, and vulnerabilities. Emotional and behavioral limitations will be reexamined. Certain goals that may previously have been judged as unattainable (not on the map) may now be seen as possible. Conversely, through repeated reality testing, unrealistic expectations are modified to become more reasonable and hence more likely to be satisfied. Often, patients need repeated confirmation that making changes can be difficult, painful, and slow but worth it in the long run.

STARTING WHERE THE PATIENT IS

Before discussing specific psychotherapeutic techniques, we would like to review two theoretical areas as background for understanding the process of the potential for patients to change their outlooks. Our focus will be on the importance of language in the creation of reality and the sense of self-efficacy.

Language and the Story

From birth onward we are bombarded with an overwhelming number of stimuli. In order to process information effectively, we tend to organize it in specific ways, lumping experiences that appear to be similar and creating rules and categories. All information about the world gets processed through our various senses: visual, auditory, and kinesthetic. In attending to the world, each of us chooses a predominant sense and communicates this in the descriptive language we use. The visually oriented person will "see what you mean," the auditory dominant person will "hear you," and the kinesthetic person will "feel" that he or she understands. Successful therapists automatically respond in the same mode as the patient.

In *The Structure of Magic*,[13] Bandler and Grinder, the founders of neurolinguistic programming (NLP), describe the process people use to record their experiences and create their maps (or stories). The basic premise is that there is a major difference between the actual world and our experience of it. Each of us creates a mental representation (story or map) of the world based on our experience. This representation subsequently governs our behavior. Since no two people have identical experiences, we all have different maps of the world.

Why is it that some people are able to respond creatively and cope productively with most of life's problems, whereas other people generally perceive few options in any situation? The second group seems to be using an impoverished map. In the face of the multifaceted, rich, and complex world we inhabit, Bandler and Grinder wondered how people maintained such limited models, even when they caused so much pain. The linguists went on to describe three perceptual mechanisms that block growth and prevent the integration of new experience: generalization, deletion, and distortion.

The overwhelming amount of information received every second by our senses must be sorted into manageable categories. Generalization is necessary for organizing information and coping with the world. Generalizing from the experience of being burned to refrain from touching a hot stove has survival value, but generalizing that all stoves are dangerous and must be avoided is dysfunctional. Having been discouraged from expressing negative feelings as a child, a person may generalize that it is bad to express any feelings. This may further generalize to the person thinking that simply having feelings is bad.

Based on early generalizations, people delete (i.e., selectively filter out) experiences that counter their established views. For example, people block themselves from hearing messages of caring that conflict with their generalizations of being unlovable. People who think of themselves as stupid will not be able to hear comments that attest to their intelligence. They will question the other's motive and accuracy of perception. Hence, we recommend the clinician say, "My, that was a difficult problem," instead of "Gee, you did that well."

The third modeling process involves distortion of sensory data to conform to preexisting notions. People hear and see what they expect to hear and see. Given a variety of experiences, people notice only those aspects that confirm their established sense of themselves and the universe. This results in their personal creation of their map, their story, or, as currently labeled, their "schema."

The process of therapy challenges the generalizations, deletions, and distortions inherent in the patient's experience of reality and thereby introduces changes into the patient's model of the world. Using cognitive therapy the clinician directly confronts these issues by challenging the generalizations, filtering (deletions) and magnifying, or personalizing (distortions) in a patient's story.

Making a Therapeutic Intervention

For the primary care practitioner what is important to remember is that language is used to organize the story about what is happening in the world and how that makes the patient feel. Language affects how the patient represents past experiences in the present, including assumed rules concerning what behaviors are acceptable and what behaviors are not acceptable. Language also structures what patients tell themselves about the future and what is likely to happen. Language is also the medium for making corrections in the story. That's what makes the practitioner's words so powerful.

It is useful to challenge generalizations and absolutes, such as always, never, everyone, and no one. For example in response to the patient, the practitioner might say, "You're absolutely *always* in pain?" "*No one* has ever accepted your ideas?" "You've *never* done anything right?" "*Everyone* is smarter than you are. Really? *Everyone?*"

Deletions are exhibited through leaving gaps in expressions. In challenging deletions, it is useful to get patients to specify missing information. When a patient says, "I'm afraid," the practitioner must respond, "Of *what* specifically are you afraid?" The response to "I'm not good enough" is "In *what way* are you not good enough?" or "Specifically, *for what* are you not good enough?" Another possible challenge would be "*How good* is good enough?" Deletions can also manifest as recognition of only the negative aspects of a situation, evaluation or otherwise positive experience.

Distortions occur not only when patients magnify potential threats, hazards or poor performance, but also when patients change verbs into nouns, such as "relating" to "relationship" or "deciding" to "decision." Bandler and Grinder point out that when we turn a "process" into an "event," which is then seen as unchangeable, this is limiting, guilt-producing, and destructive:

> Patient: "I really regret my decision."
>
> The response: "What stops you from changing your mind now?"
>
> Patient: "My relationship is a disaster."
>
> The response: "Is there a way you can respond to your partner in a more constructive way?"

In challenging models, the practitioner questions not only absolutes but also imposed limits (the can'ts, shoulds, musts, and impossibilities – "Why not?") and imposed values (rights, wrongs, "goods," and "bads") and in the process helps the patient to create a richer representation of possibilities.

The Power Inherent in the Word or Concept of "yet"

Helping patients to edit their stories does not have to be time-consuming or complicated. For instance, the word "yet" is a very efficient therapeutic tool. When a patient makes a statement about his or her inability to do something, the practitioner can counter, "You have not been able to do that yet!" or "Up to now, this has been difficult for you." These statements imply that this is not a permanent situation. This simple intervention is actually psychotherapy. It has the potential to change the patient's view of what is possible. The same technique can be used to respond to statements when patients complain that they "always" have a certain difficulty. The response: "Yes, that has been your experience so far. You have not solved it yet." The take home message for the patient is that the practitioner believes that the patient is capable of achieving a particular goal. This can directly affect the patient's sense of self-efficacy.

The Sense of Self-efficacy

In treating dysfunctional behavior we have found that cognitive processes, which we term "stories," determine and maintain habitual functioning. Successful change depends on changing habits and is performance-oriented, meaning that it relates to doing something. Albert Bandura[14] first postulated the concept of self-efficacy as a way to explain the reciprocal relationship between performance and the cognitive assessment of the likelihood of success. Self-efficacy refers to people's beliefs in their ability to succeed at something. These beliefs are based on past performance, vicarious experience, physiological and psychological states, and feedback regarding the current performance. Self-efficacy determines whether behavior is initiated, the amount of effort that is expended, and how long that effort is sustained when obstacles or adverse reactions are experienced.

The concept of self-efficacy is very useful for understanding and predicting behavior and also for providing a strategy to induce change. A diverse and rapidly expanding medical literature documents the importance of self-efficacy. This includes the relationship between self-efficacy and chronic obstructive pulmonary disease (COPD),[15] return to work after angioplasty,[16] mediating disability related to chronic pain,[17] recovery from orthopedic surgery,[18] quality of life of cancer patients,[19] maintaining physical and role functioning in coronary heart disease[20] and treatment for chronic alcoholism,[21] to mention only a few. The bottom line is that patients' predictions of what they will do are the most reliable indicators of what will transpire. If patients think that they are able to do something, they will try. If they fail at first, they will continue to try because they believe it is only a question of time until they will succeed. Conversely, if patients have a low sense of self-efficacy and do not expect to be able to succeed, they may or may not try, their effort will be limited, and on encountering difficulties, their tendency will be to give up since they expect to fail anyway.

There is little sense in prescribing medication to help patients stop smoking until those patients believe they can kick the habit, redefine themselves as nonsmokers, and develop healthy activities to substitute for the smoking urge. The sense of self-efficacy is not just an estimate of potential performance based on perceptions of past accomplishment but is directly instrumental in enhancing performance.[22]

Bandura's work is valuable because it points to mechanisms that can positively affect the sense of self-efficacy. These include structuring successes to modify the efficacy expectation. This can be done by setting achievable goals and aiming for small wins as will be discussed later. Self-efficacy can also be affected by providing vicarious experiences such as evidence that others in similar circumstances have been successful. Creating supportive environments and encouraging trial and error learning is also effective. Finally, practitioners can use verbal persuasion to change patients' views of the task or themselves by focusing on past successes or using the word "yet." In essence, CBT can be used to affect the sense of self-efficacy.

The Power of Positive Illusions

Traditional concepts of mental health have proposed that well-adjusted individuals have a relatively accurate perception of themselves and their ability to control important aspects of their lives. There is now an impressive body of literature that suggests that having positive illusions about the self, personal control, and the future not only enhances performance, but also results in a wide range of positive mental health outcomes.[23] This, too, can be seen as evidence that people's stories become self-fulfilling prophecies.

In summary, positive information that the practitioner provides about the patient or about a task (that the patient has just not been successful *yet*) may affect the patient's sense of self-efficacy and encourage the patient to engage in beneficial behavior change. The resulting positive outcome then further enhances the patient's sense of self-efficacy. Subsequently, the patient's story about what can be accomplished changes. The therapeutic intervention has been successful.

USEFUL TECHNIQUES FROM A VARIETY OF SOURCES

Having outlined the major generic therapeutic components common to all psychotherapeutic interventions and sketched some interesting models that explain the mechanisms involved in patient's limited outlooks, we will now focus on therapeutic pearls from a variety of orientations. There are clearly some techniques that are more effective than others, some that are easier to learn than others, and some that lend themselves more comfortably to a therapeutic encounter within a 15-minute framework.

Psychodynamics in Brief

In general, people are simpler than insight schools imply, but more complex than behavioral models suggest. By simpler we mean that a limited number of supportive techniques are highly effective, and by complex we mean that people's reactions are determined by a multitude of factors both in and out of awareness.

The unique contribution of psychodynamic theories is pointing out the hidden agendas that pervade interpersonal relationships. Maladaptive personal responses, influenced by past experiences, are projected onto current relationships. Some of this process is purely symbolic and unconscious, and some is within the awareness of the patient. The way patients define themselves as loving or hateful, competent or inadequate, is an ongoing process, a story that they are telling themselves based on judgments they have made over time. Since much of this behavior is demonstrated in relation to the practitioner, an opportunity is created to bring these dynamics into focus and to challenge the accuracy of the story.

The Healing Relationship

From Carl Rogers we have learned the value of relating to patients in a non-possessive, accepting way and expressing our caring by providing accurate empathy.[24] The accepting practitioner creates a safe environment that facilitates the exploration of various possibilities for change.

Empathic understanding is communicated to the patient through techniques of active and accurate listening. This is demonstrated by first listening to the story without interrupting for one or two minutes and then paraphrasing, summarizing, reflecting feelings, and responding authentically. According to Rogers, however, these techniques are relatively unimportant except as a channel for communicating positive regard and accurate empathy.[24] Sometimes, it takes a while for the patient to receive the communication. Repeated visits to a primary care practitioner create the perfect medium to allow the message to sink in.

Behavioral Therapies

The evolution of behavioral therapies since Bandura[25] first conceptualized psychotherapy as a learning process in the early 1960s has been phenomenal. In a review of 252 empirical studies of psychotherapy over three decades, the 1960s, 1970s and 1980s, H. Omer and R. Dar[26] document the striking evolution away from theory-guided research to pragmatic, clinically oriented research.

The popularity of behavioral approaches to therapy can be attributed to their utility in helping patients find solutions to their problems in living. Relaxation, desensitization, visualization, assertiveness training, and biofeedback are all part of CBT and all stem from behaviorism. Patients practice and learn new ways to manage themselves, their anxiety, and their behavior. Research has repeatedly demonstrated that thinking is a behavior that can be modified and that modes of thinking affect the origin, maintenance, and change process related to various human problems.[27] People are often not aware that how they think about a situation directly influences how they feel about it. Albert Ellis pointed out that when we think about our goals, even the process of planning steps that we can take to further these goals results in positive feelings.[28]

Ellis also underscored the importance of identifying the rigid, dogmatic, and powerful demands and commands that constitute the irrational beliefs most of us hold regarding the way the world is supposed to be. He pointed out that it is important to dispute statements such as "It's awful" (meaning totally bad or more than bad!) or "I can't bear it" (meaning survive or be happy at all!).[27] Beck and Young[29] have successfully used these techniques to help severely depressed persons counter the negative thoughts and evaluations of self, others, and circumstances that trigger and maintain depressive syndromes. Schema-focused therapy[30] incorporates cognitive, experiential, interpersonal, and behavioral techniques for working with patients with personality disorders and other difficult chronic syndromes. David Barlow[31] combines cognitive techniques with various forms of relaxation training in the treatment of panic and other anxiety disorders. This is the essence of CBT. These techniques are powerful, especially when promoted and initiated by a primary care practitioner.

Relaxation Training

Relaxation techniques are designed to help individuals cope with their stress and anxiety and the accompanying physical symptoms. It is not difficult to teach patients techniques to help them relax. It also does not take a great deal of time. These techniques can be learned easily during a 15-minute visit. It does, however, require patients to practice the techniques daily, for periods of perhaps 10 minutes, for at least two weeks. Practitioners must explain to patients that the experience of anxiety or stress is mutually exclusive with relaxation. When stressed, patients will take shallow and rapid breaths, tense their muscles, and experience racing, negative thoughts. To physically control stress and anxiety, patients are instructed to focus on their breathing, exhaling completely while trying to push their stomachs into their spines. When they inhale they will fill their lungs all the way to their diaphragms. This is called "belly breathing." It results in a relaxation response. When patients focus their attention on their breathing, it puts them in control of this previously automatic behavior, and becomes a powerful antidote to stress. Ideally, patients will do this for a few minutes several times each day, but breathing techniques can be used as needed during periods of stress. As previously stated, "belly breathing," deep from the diaphragm, requires a certain amount of practice to become comfortable and ultimately automatic.

Patients can also be instructed to intentionally relax their muscles. It is good to start by having patients alternately tense and relax specific muscle groups in order to help them distinguish between tension and relaxation. They can focus on hands, arms, and shoulders; then the face and neck; followed by feet, legs, and buttocks; and finally chest and abdomen. After all muscle groups have been completely relaxed, patients will enjoy relief of pain and stress. Once they have learned to control their breathing and relax their muscles, patients can be instructed to focus on specific positive thoughts. After a little more practice, they can learn to visualize and create mental representations of healing experiences.

These techniques can be used to countermand a variety of symptoms from anxiety, headaches, and general tension to chronic pain. They can be thought of as "behavioral aspirin," powerful therapeutic interventions with no negative side effects. They empower patients and give them positive choices. These instructions can be reinforced by patient education handouts or by recommending self-help books, some of which are listed in Appendix B. However, the power of the intervention derives from being taught and monitored by a primary care practitioner with the stated assurance about its efficacy. These relaxation techniques defined as "behavioral therapies" are subsumed under CBT.

Narrative Therapy

A promising modality, using specific cognitive techniques, that is gaining increased recognition is narrative therapy.[32] Michael White, an Australian practitioner, built on the notion that all our knowledge of the world is carried through mental maps of external reality. Since no map includes every detail of the territory, events that do not make it onto the map do not exist in that map's world of meaning. White suggested that "a story is map that extends through time."[32] This postmodern, narrative, social constructionist worldview offers useful ideas about how power, knowledge, and "truth" are negotiated in families and larger cultures. The basic theses of this worldview include the following:

1. realities are socially constructed
2. realities are constituted through language
3. realities are organized and maintained through narrative
4. there are no essential truths.

Michael White introduced the technique of "relative influence questioning" as a way to separate patients from their problems and help them to invent more positive stories. Patients are asked to map the influence of a particular problem on their lives and their relationships and then to map their influence on the life of the problem. Rather than being the problem, people have relationships with the problem. They are then invited to speculate about changing the future. What would their life be like if they did not have this problem? Would this be an improved experience? How would they act? How would they feel? Was there a time in the past when they felt that way? What did they do differently at the time? Then they are asked to link the two episodes. This is followed by questions that extend the story into the future. Narrative therapists ask questions to generate experiences rather than to gather information. White suggests that when we ask questions, we are generating possible versions of a life. Experience is colored and shaped by the meaning people give it. How people will attend to the experience is related to the stories people are living. Narrative therapy makes a shift from gathering information to generating experience. We contend that questions intentionally asked by primary care practitioners can be powerful therapeutic interventions. Questions posed do not necessarily have to be answered during a session but can be left as unfinished business for the patient to consider.

White distinguishes five specific kinds of questions. "Deconstruction questions" unpack the story and help people to see different perspectives. They are invited to distinguish particular beliefs, practices, feelings, and attitudes. Practitioners might ask about history, context, effects or results, interrelationships, and tactics or strategies. "Opening space questions" inquire about unique outcomes. They probe hypothetical experiences and different contexts and time frames; for example, "In what situations do you have a different reaction?" "Preference questions" look at whether the patient would be better or worse off without the problem. "Story development questions" invite people to relate the process and details of an experience and to connect it to a time frame, a particular context, and other people. "Meaning questions" explore patients' motivations, hopes, goals, values, and beliefs. Story development and meaning questions help in story reconstruction. These techniques are not only practical, but also highly effective and can be used to explore patients' stories about their health and disease, as well as social functioning.

Expecting Patient Follow-through

According to William Glasser MD, patients develop many symptoms and engage in irresponsible behavior because they are not controlling their lives and because they choose not to feel the painful emotions triggered by the situation.[33] Often, these painful emotions are converted to physical pain in various parts of the body. Glasser says that what we label as mental illness, regardless of the causation, are the hundreds of ways people choose to behave when they are unable to satisfy their innate needs for love and power to the extent they want. When patients do not feel worthwhile to themselves and others (competent) or loved (connected) they need the warmth, kindness, and strength of a practitioner who will support them while at the same time holding them responsible for changing their behavior. Using Glasser's approach, the practitioner acts as a coach, encouraging the patient to focus on current behavior, evaluate that behavior, and plan alternate (more constructive) behavior. The crux of this therapy is that the patient is expected to take responsibility for follow-through. No excuses are accepted. If a plan is reasonable, there are no excuses. At the same time, there is no punishment. Instead, there is consistent insistence that commitments be honored. Patients become aware that there are consequences in real life for poor choices and failure to carry out commitments. The therapeutic relationship, however, remains one of respect, caring, and involvement through mutual setting of reasonable expectations and monitoring of results. These interventions combine the best of theory and pragmatic application, and they really work.

DETERMINING LEVELS OF INVOLVEMENT IN PRACTICE: PLISSIT

Any encounter that inspires the patient's hopes for improvement, be it one visit or several, is therapeutic. For the primary care practitioner, however, it is useful to have a protocol to guide the level of intervention. A mechanistic, but practical and effective hierarchical system was first introduced by J.S. Annon in the context of sex therapy.[34] This four-step process triggered by the acronym "PLISSIT" is easily remembered and simple to apply.

In a potentially therapeutic situation, where the patient is concerned with certain reactions to a particular situation, the levels of intervention go from permission giving, to offering limited information, to specific suggestions, to a contract for intensive therapy.

P Stands for Permission

Regardless of what else transpires in the therapeutic session, it is always appropriate to give patients permission to feel what they feel. This simple intervention does more to restore patients' equilibrium than almost anything else the practitioner can do. When patients become aware that the world or other people are not as they want them to be or that they are not handling situations as well as they want to, they feel badly. When the practitioner reassures the patient that the reaction being experienced is normal under the circumstances, the patient feels better. The patient recognizes that it is O.K. to be depressed and does not have to be depressed about being depressed or feel anxious about being anxious. When a patient relates that he lost his temper and yelled at his wife, the practitioner can assure him it is normal to get angry, especially when one is under stress. It happens. However, the patient does need to let his wife know that he is sorry.

It is important to give people permission to feel the way they feel, because if they could feel any other way, at a particular time, they would. The practitioner's understanding and acceptance make the patient feel more comfortable with the emotional state being experienced.

LI Stands for Limited Information

The second level of intervention is to provide a small amount of essential information to explain the emotional state being experienced. This helps patients set realistic expectations for themselves and others. For example, a patient in a situation of crisis is told that in general, when people experience great amounts of stress they react by feeling overwhelmed, confused, and less capable of making decisions or solving problems; can't remember recently learned information; have trouble sleeping; and so on. This normalization helps get the patient off *tilt*. When practitioners make this kind of ubiquitous statement, patients feel as though given the circumstances their reactions are appropriate after all. Information processing is a high-order coping skill. By offering accurate and pertinent information, in small enough amounts for patients to assimilate, the practitioner is being highly supportive.

SS Stands for Specific Suggestions

Specific suggestions can be given to the patient to examine options, pose questions, visit a particular website to get information, talk to friends, get into a self-help group, take time out, keep a journal, or employ any other specific strategy that helps to engage the patient's healthy functioning self and promote constructive coping behavior. These suggestions must be tailored to fit into the patient's current lifestyle and not present one more overwhelming demand. Often it is useful to ask the patient, "What one thing could you do that would make you feel a little better?" "What can you do to get more information before you make that important decision?" The practitioner's involvement and confidence that the patient is competent and can take control of the situation, foster this behavior in the patient.

IT Stands for Intensive Therapy

Intensive therapy as it applies to the primary care setting implies that the practitioner makes a commitment to work with the patient over time. Appointments are scheduled, and the practitioner contracts to offer support for the patient for a specific time in order to resolve a particular life problem. By engaging in a therapeutic contract with the patient, all five criteria specified in the section on common psychotherapeutic elements are satisfied. Positive expectations that help is forthcoming are instigated. A therapeutic relationship is established. The patient receives an external perspective on the problem. Corrective experiences are encouraged, and the patient is given the opportunity to test reality repeatedly. The practitioner connects with the patient and helps to further his or her sense of competency.

SUMMARY

Practical therapeutic interventions treat emotional, behavioral, personality, or psychiatric disorders, primarily through communication with the patient. Psychotherapy helps patients edit their "stories." Therapeutic goals are generic (making patients feel better and less overwhelmed), incremental (manageable), and specific (making patients feel competent and connected to others).

Supportive therapy focuses on the patients' strengths, whereas exploratory therapy traces the etiology of feelings. It is more important to help patients change their reactions than to understand their source. Common elements among psychotherapeutic techniques include (1) the expectation of receiving help, (2) participation in a therapeutic relationship, (3) obtaining an external perspective on problems, (4) the encouragement of corrective experiences, and (5) the opportunity to test reality repeatedly.

Language is used to record and classify our perceptual experience of the world. Through processes of generalization, deletion, and distortion, people build impoverished "maps," or models of the world, which then limit their perceived options. The therapeutic process challenges these generalizations, deletions, and distortions in order to create a richer representation of possibilities. Cognitive techniques can help patients attend to and modify these unproductive thought patterns. People's sense of self-efficacy is directly related to outcomes. Behavior therapies underscore the importance of human learning in the process of modifying behavior. Cognitive therapy is based on modifying "irrational" beliefs that affect how people react to situations. The word "yet" is a powerful therapeutic tool since it implies that change is pending. It is not difficult to teach patients the techniques of belly breathing and muscle relaxation to manage stress and anxiety. It also does not take a great deal of time. Narrative therapy uses focused questions to help patients reconstruct reality.

Through the creation of a warm and understanding relationship, a practitioner encourages patients to accept responsibility for their behavior.

The acronym "PLISSIT" can be used to structure levels of intervention, from simple permission giving, to offering limited information, making specific suggestions, or entering into a contract for intensive therapy.

References

1. Gaudiano BA. Cognitive-behavioural therapies: achievements and challenges. *Evid Based Ment Health*. 2008; **11**: 5–7.
2. Frank JD. *Persuasion and Healing*. Rev. ed. Baltimore: Johns Hopkins; 1973.
3. Welwood J. *Journey of the Heart: intimate relationship and the path of love*. New York: HarperCollins; 1990. p. 25.
4. Leichsenring F. Comparative effects of short-term psychodynamic psychotherapy and cognitive-behavioral therapy in depression: a meta-analytic approach. *Clin Psychol Rev*. 2001; **21**: 401–19.
5. Haug TT, Mykletun A, Dahl AA. The association between anxiety, depression, and somatic symptoms in a large population: the HUNT-II Study. *Psychosom Med*. 2004; **66**: 845–51.
6. Rodin J. Aging and health: effects of the sense of control. *Science*. 1986; **233**: 1271–5.
7. Schaubroeck J, Jones JR, Xie JL. Individual differences in utilizing control to cope with job demands: effects on susceptibility to infectious disease. *J Appl Psychol*. 2001; **86**(2): 265–78.
8. Miller GE, Cohen S. Psychological interventions and the immune system: a meta-analytic review and critique. *Health Psychol*. 2001; **20**: 47–63.
9. Frank JD. Therapeutic components. In: Myers JM, (ed.) *Cures by Psychotherapy: what effects change?* New York: Praeger; 1984.
10. Watzlawick P, Weakland JH, Fisch R. *Change: principles of problem formation and problem resolution*. New York: W.W. Norton & Co.; 1974.
11. Goldfried MR. Rapproachment of psychotherapies. *J Hum Psych*. 1983; **23**: 97–107.
12. Frank JD. Psychotherapy: the restoration of morale. *Am J Psychiatry*. 1974; **131**: 271–4.
13. Bandler R, Grinder J. *The Structure of Magic. I. A Book about Language and Therapy*. Palo Alto, CA: Science and Behavior Books; 1975.
14. Bandura A. Self-efficacy: toward a unifying theory of behavioral change. *Psychol Rev*. 1977; **84**(2): 191–215.
15. Wigal JK, Creer TL, Kotses H. The COPD Self-Efficacy Scale. *Chest*. 1991; **99**(5): 1193–6.
16. Newman S. Engaging patients in managing their cardiovascular health. *Heart*. 2004; **90**(Suppl. 4): 9–13.
17. Arnstein P. The mediation of disability by self-efficacy in different samples of chronic pain patients. *Disabil Rehabil*. 2000; **22**(17): 794–801.
18. Waldrop D, Lightsey OR, Ethington CA, *et al*. Self-efficacy, optimism, health competence, and recovery from orthopedic surgery. *J Couns Psychol*. 2001; **48**(2): 233–8.
19. Cunningham AJ, Lockwood GA, Cunningham JA. A relationship between perceived self-efficacy and quality of life in cancer patients. *Patient Educ Couns*. 1991; **17**(1): 71–8.

20. Sullivan M, LaCroix AZ, Russo J, *et al.* Self-efficacy and self-reported functional status in coronary heart disease: a six-month prospective study. *Psychosom Med.* 1998; **60**(4): 473–8.

21. Ilgen M, Tiet Q, Finne J, *et al.* Self-efficacy, therapeutic alliance, and alcohol-use disorder treatment outcomes. *J Stud Alcohol.* 2006; **67**(3): 465–72.

22. Bandura A. Recycling misconceptions of perceived self-efficacy. *Cognit Ther Res.* 1984; **8**: 231–55.

23. Taylor SE, Kemeny ME, Reed GM, *et al.* Psychological resources, positive illusions and health. *Am Psychol.* 2000, **55**(1): 99–109.

24. Rogers C. The necessary and sufficient conditions of therapeutic personality change. *J Consult Psychol.* 1957; **21**: 95–103.

25. Bandura A. Psychotherapy as a learning process. *Psychol Bull.* 1961; **58**: 143–59.

26. Omer H, Dar R. Changing trends in three decades of psychotherapy research: the flight from theory into pragmatics. *J Consult Clin Psych.* 1992; **60**: 88–93.

27. Ellis A. The revised ABC's of rational-emotive therapy (RET). *J Rational-Emotive & Cog-Behav Ther.* 1991; **9**: 139–72.

28. Ellis, op. cit. p. 144.

29. Beck AT, Young JE. Depression. In: Barlow DH, (ed.) *Clinical Handbook of Psychological Disorders.* New York: Guilford Press; 1985. pp. 206–44.

30. Young JD. *Cognitive Therapy for Personality Disorders: a schema-focused approach,* 3rd ed. Sarasota, Fla.: Professional Resource Press; 1999.

31. Barlow DH. Cognitive-behavioral therapy for panic disorder: current status. *J Clin Psychiatry.* 1997; **58**(Suppl. 2): 32–6.

32. Freedan J, Combs G. *Narrative Therapy: the social construction of preferred realities.* New York: W.W. Norton & Co.; 1996.

33. Glasser W. *Reality Therapy in Action.* New York: HarperCollins; 2000.

34. Annon JS. *Behavioral Treatment of Sexual Problems: brief therapy.* New York: Harper & Row; 1976.

CHAPTER 4

Starting with the BATHE Technique

Because the body-mind is essentially one, and patients' responses to stress can precipitate an office visit, are we really suggesting that the patient's psychological needs should be addressed during *every* patient visit? Actually, we are! Of course, there are exceptions. If a patient is profusely bleeding, is comatose or in acute pain from an ongoing cardiac event, you might want to postpone this inquiry, but it is not necessarily irrelevant. If a patient appears psychotic or becomes hostile or defensive, obviously it is best to focus directly on the patient's stated needs. However, just as there are recognized advantages to periodic health screening from a biomedical perspective, many benefits accrue from assessing a patient's emotional and social status as part of each visit. Moreover, it is not a difficult task to obtain psychosocial data in an efficient and effective manner. The BATHE technique is extremely versatile and can be used for both opening and closing the psychosocial inquiry, to access important information for the clinician in a variety of situations, and to provide support for the patient.

Imagine a reasonably sensitive and specific screening test that takes about one minute, uses no supplies, is noninvasive, has no harmful side effects, and is generally acceptable to patients. Imagine further that this test may pick up potentially serious problems in an early, treatable stage and can be expected to yield *at least* 30% positive results.[1,2] Finally, imagine that use of the test might provide beneficial results for the patient, that completing the test might actually be therapeutic. Would you use such a test regularly? We think so.

Another benefit of using the BATHE technique is that exploration of the psychosocial aspects of the patient's problems provides an additional level of complexity of treatment and adds value and quality to the services delivered. In any case, use of the test is likely to improve clinical outcomes as well as increasing patient satisfaction.[3]

OPENING THE THERAPEUTIC INQUIRY

Primary care practitioners have a unique opportunity to address the emotional needs of their patients, but regardless of their importance, these needs must be handled in a time-effective manner. The psychosocial aspect of patients' problems must be effectively addressed within the regular 10 or 15-minute medical visit. The therapeutic goal is to help patients reorganize some small aspect of their self-concept or behavior in a more comfortable, productive, or, at minimum, less destructive manner. The healing grows out of the established practitioner-patient relationship.

The specific treatment attempts to modify patients' images of themselves, their problems, and their options by adjusting their *assumptive world view*, the story they tell themselves about the way things are. As we have said earlier, good interviewing techniques, a caring manner, and genuine interest demonstrated by paying serious attention to the patient's problems pave the way toward establishing a therapeutic milieu. In the process, patients feel supported and less stressed and able to raise their level of self-esteem as well as reengage their healthier coping styles.[4] Not only does the practitioner gain a healthier and more reasonable patient, but using this technique, with its small investment of time during each patient visit, may save the practitioner a tremendous amount of time in some future encounter. If a patient's psychological needs are not addressed and are allowed to compound over time, they can present as a monumental problem that will overextend the practitioner's resources at a subsequent visit.

Determining the Context of the Visit

Optimally, every physical complaint or office visit should be seen in the context of the patient's and his or her family's total life situation. This means that in addition to descriptions of presenting symptoms, which may well represent a response to situational stress, the practitioner must determine what is going on in the patient's life as part of the history of the present illness.

Nowadays, most primary care practitioners organize their charts around the problem-oriented medical record.[5] Problems are listed and notes are arranged in *SOAP* fashion. Most practitioners are familiar with this system, which classifies progress notes into subjective, objective, assessment, and plan elements. In order to understand patients' problems in the context of their total life situations, primary care practitioners need a larger concept of *SOAP*.[6] The total package of patient assessment requires determination of the background situation, the patient's affect, what is most troubling for the patient, and how the patient is handling things. To achieve closure, this assessment needs to be followed by an empathic response.[7]

THE BATHE TECHNIQUE

TABLE 4.1

B	–	BACKGROUND: What is going on in your life?
A	–	AFFECT: How do you feel about that?
T	–	TROUBLE: What troubles you the most?
H	–	HANDLING: How are you handling that?
E	–	EMPATHY: That must be very difficult.

The acronym "BATHE" connotes memory jogs for the protocol to determine the context of the visit. It can also be viewed as an informal screening test for emotional problems.

B stands for background. A simple question, "What is going on in your life?" will elicit the context of the patient's visit. Alternative opening questions can take the form of "Tell me what's been happening since I saw you last?" It is useful to connect with patients in this personal way at each visit.

A stands for affect (the feeling state). "How do you feel about that?", "How does that make you feel?" or "What's your mood?" allows the patient to report the current feeling state.

T stands for trouble. "What about the situation troubles you the most?" helps both the practitioner and the patient focus on the subjective meaning of the situation.

H stands for handling. "How are you handling that?" gives an assessment of functioning.

E stands for empathy. A response such as "That must be very difficult for you" legitimizes the patient's reaction.

The empathic response reassures the patient that the practitioner has understood the situation and accepts the patient's response as reasonable, given the circumstances. BATHE is all that is minimally required to make the patient feel supported. At the same time, the technique will also enable the practitioner to identify depression, anxiety, or other disturbing symptoms. Ideally the BATHE technique will be employed early in the interview after the chief complaint and history of the presenting illness have been explored. BATHE may help determine why the patient is here now. It is useful to discuss each of the elements of BATHE separately.

"B" Stands for Background

The opening question of the BATHE sequence addresses what has been happening in the patient's life. If the patient's chief complaint concerns a problem that started perhaps two weeks previously, then the question becomes "What was going on in your life about that time?" We do not recommend asking if there was anything "new" or particularly stressful. Yes or no questions do not supply many bits of information, and there may or may not have been a major stress. Furthermore, daily hassles are often more detrimental to a patient's sense of well-being than a new major stressful event.[8]

Although it is useful to determine what might have precipitated the patient's problem, the background question is probably the least important of the BATHE questions. Even with a positive response concerning a specific problematic situation, it is best not to encourage patients to tell you more about the situation; if you do, they will. And that will use up precious time without necessarily leading to any useful outcome. The situation will not change. You simply want to understand the patient's response. Further discussion of dealing with the "run-on" patient can be found in Chapter 6.

Often, patients will deny any particular stress. They may say that nothing has been going on – or perhaps just the "same old thing." Regardless of the patient's answer to the first question, about what is going on, it is effective to go directly to the next question: "How does that make you feel?"

"A" is for Affect

Asking patients how they feel about what is going on in their lives serves several important functions. In the first place it satisfies one of the critical requirements of the patient-centered interview,[9] addressing the patient's emotional response. Often patients are not in touch with their emotional response. Illness behavior is a universal mechanism used by people with psychological disturbance to express their distress and seek medical care.[10-12] Helping patients get in touch with and express their feelings directly is highly therapeutic. Once expressed, feelings do not have to be "somatized." When patients are labeling their feelings, they should be encouraged to use adjectives such as mad, glad, sad, disappointed, frustrated, devastated, or guilty. Sometimes patients will use the phrase "I feel that" to express a judgment. Any time you can substitute the phrase "I feel" for the words "I think" – that is not a feeling. Feelings are whatever feelings are. They are neither good nor bad, but that individual's response to the particular situation. Feelings do not need to be justified or explained; they just have to be accepted. Many people are uncomfortable with the feelings they have. It is highly therapeutic to give people permission to feel the way they feel. In the BATHE sequence, the practitioner uses attentive listening and body language to make the patient feel accepted. If the patient is having a problem labeling a feeling, the practitioner may wish to suggest that under similar circumstances many people would feel angry, frustrated, overwhelmed, or whatever an appropriate response might be.

"T" Stands for Trouble

This is the most important of the BATHE questions. "What about the situation troubles you the most?" helps the patient to get in touch with the meaning of the situation. This question generally requires the patient to stop and think. Many people are not particularly self-reflecting without some coaching. It has been our experience that confronted with the question "What about that troubles you?", after pausing and focusing, patients often have an "Aha!" reaction and realize something that had been out of their awareness until that time.

Practitioners are often surprised by the answers that this question elicits since people have unique reactions to common situational circumstances. Since what is most troubling about the situation constitutes the definition of the problem, arriving at some constructive solution now becomes possible. When patients relate some positive event in their lives and a positive feeling to accompany it, it is still useful to ask whether anything about the situation troubles the patient, since ambivalence is a common human experience. Posing this question allows the patient to express reservations that may or may not be significant but need to be acknowledged.

"H" Stands for Handling

This question can be used in different ways. Asking "How are you handling that?" gives the practitioner valuable information about possibly destructive behaviors that the patient may be using to cope. Perhaps the patient is abusing alcohol, binge eating or fighting with significant others. Often the patient will reply, "not very well" and list some of the symptoms that prompted the office visit and then wonder if perhaps the situation precipitated those reactions. In other words, the (Socratic) questioning allows patients to get in touch with answers they already have but are not aware of.

Sometimes it is more efficacious to ask, "How could you handle that?" This intervention empowers patients to arrive at solutions they may not have considered previously. The implication is that they are capable of dealing with the situation constructively. Later chapters will discuss a variety of tasks that can be assigned as homework to help patients come to positive resolution of their problems.

"E" Stands for Empathy

It is crucial that practitioners finish the BATHE sequence with a statement that demonstrates understanding and empathy. Acknowledging the difficulty of the situation, the fact that the patient is doing the best that can be expected under the circumstances or that this is obviously very painful, validates the patient's experience and makes him or her feel competent and connected in a positive way to the practitioner. This acknowledgment provides effective psychological support. It also closes the inquiry and allows the practitioner to move back to the physical aspects of the patient's problem.

When the BATHE technique is used effectively, situational factors are identified, feelings are validated, meaning is assessed, a plan is made, and psychological support is provided. Nothing further is required. The intervention is complete. The whole interaction usually takes less than one minute.

WHAT IS THE BEST TIME TO BATHE?

When practitioners apply the BATHE technique as part of the history of present illness (HPI) in the interview, an effective and efficient therapeutic intervention is structured into every patient encounter. The context of the visit has been incorporated into the session, patients' emotional reactions are addressed, and there is closure. A basic screening for anxiety or depressive disorders has also been accomplished. Sometimes there may not be a problem, but having the opportunity for social intercourse is still gratifying for the patient.[13,14] Most of the time, patients reveal some ongoing concern. Often the patient feels better immediately after completion of the BATHE protocol, having become aware of the underlying issue that makes a situation problematic. The practitioner's interest and empathic response make the patient feel connected. Being able to sort out the problem and exploring the notion of "handling it" makes the patient feel more competent. The practitioner then proceeds with further medical history and the appropriate physical examination. When the routine BATHE interaction uncovers a serious problem, additional support and/or provision for follow-up or referral can be addressed with the assessment and plan part of the visit, as shown by the following example:

A 34-year-old woman, who had been a patient at the family practice center for about one year, presented in the office complaining about a vaginal discharge. She appeared to be quite agitated. Dr. W., in his second year of training at the time, inquired about what was going on in her life. The patient started to cry. She reached for the box of tissues on the desk. The physician waited quietly for her to answer his question.

"I just found out that my husband has been having an affair with my oldest sister for the past year and a half."

"How do you feel about that?" (The physician felt a little foolish. It seemed like this was an inane question to ask under the circumstances, but he really did not know what else to ask.)

Between sobs, the patient responded, "I feel angry. I have mood swings. I go up and down. I also feel depressed."

After taking several deep breaths to center himself, Dr. W. asked what about the situation troubled the patient the most. She replied, "I have two children. They are two and five, and I really don't want to be a single parent."

(The physician was surprised. He would have expected her to be most troubled because of the familial involvement, the betrayal, or the time frame.)

"How are you handling it?" was his final question.

The patient stated that she was handling things very badly. She was angry and did a lot of shouting at her husband. She also added that she was afraid that the children were starting to be affected, she was very short-tempered with them, and they really did not deserve that.

The physician was taken aback by this history. Still, he managed to respond, "That sounds like a horrendous situation. It's got to be hard for you to deal with all of that."

"Yes, it is," said the patient and visibly relaxed.

"Why don't we examine you now and find out what we can do about your vaginal discomfort," said the physician, "and then we'll talk some more and get you some help."

Patients' Understanding of Stress

Happily not all situations are as dramatic or traumatic as the above example. In our practice BATHE is used routinely and uncovers a variety of situations, more often chronic rather than acute. Our experience has been that the technique is well accepted by patients, even those coming from a variety of cultures. Once confronted by a focused question, patients are often acutely aware of the role of stress in precipitating their symptoms. Consider the following description of a visit reported by a psychology intern who had monitored the encounter over closed-circuit television:

Ms. K. is a middle-aged African-American female, a college student, who has come to the office for an initial visit. Her presenting problem is a dry scalp with associated peeling and flaking. She reports that she has been experiencing this problem for several weeks but that lately it seems to have worsened. She appears pleasant and cooperative during the discussion of her symptomatology and throughout the subsequent physical examination by the physician. However, she offers no complaints regarding situational stressors or issues of concern in her life.

When the doctor specifically *asks what was going on in the patient's life*, she responds by saying she is an older woman and is currently back in school. The physician then *asks how she feels about this*. The patient seems slightly uncomfortable disclosing her feelings and focuses instead on discussing the content of her college program. The physician listens intently for a brief while. Then he patiently *asks again how she feels about that*. Ms. K.'s shoulders appear to relax as she admits to feeling rather stressed out concerning the challenges of returning to school later in life. The physician then comments that *that must be very difficult for her*. The patient nods her head in agreement and seems relieved to have her feelings validated.

The doctor then asks *what troubles the patient the most about her situation*. The patient discloses that she finds the workload and associated stress and anxiety most disconcerting. The doctor then *inquires how she has been handling the anxiety*. At this point, the patient shares laughter with the doctor as she replies that a lot of prayers have been getting her through.

The physician acknowledges the helpfulness of prayer and then introduces the importance of exercise as a further means of reducing stress. Ms. K. reports that she used to exercise but has not lately. The doctor then explains, "The reason that I am asking about your stress is that there is a mind-body connection and often psychological issues can manifest as or exacerbate physical problems such as with your scalp." This appears to strike a responsive chord with the patient as she relates, "Oh, yes, Doctor, in fact a few years ago when I was going through a stressful divorce, I remember having similar problems with my scalp." The discussion then returns to the topic of exercise, and with the patient's eager collaboration, together they formulate a daily exercise regimen that can realistically be implemented given the rigorous demands of Ms. K.'s scholastic program.

In this situation, the physician weaves BATHE into the encounter and is able to use it to help the patient make sense of her symptoms as well as prescribing and getting agreement for an effective management plan.

SUPPORTING THE PATIENT

In Chapter 2 we defined social support as a psychological mechanism that provides positive information to the individual about his or her interaction with other people. More technically, in social science studies social support has been defined as "the sum of the social, emotional and instrumental exchanges with which the individual is involved having the subjective consequence that an individual sees him or herself as an object of continuing value in the eyes of significant others."[15] Certainly, the interaction between the patient and the practitioner involves social, emotional, and instrumental exchanges. It is obviously important that practitioners behave in such a manner that patients get the impression that they are seen as individuals who have continuing value in the eyes of the practitioner. Social support has been shown to be critical in mitigating the effects of various stressors.[16] Social support is demonstrated by engaging in one or more of the following behaviors: (1) an expression of positive affect, (2) an endorsement of the person's behavior, perception, or expressed views, (3) giving symbolic or material aid, and (4) giving the opportunity to express feelings in an accepting atmosphere.

It is clear that when practitioners incorporate BATHE into a patient visit, many of the above criteria will be satisfied. Interest and positive affect have been expressed, and feelings have been accepted. Information is gathered that helps both patient and practitioner understand the situation and the patient's reaction to it, and the diagnosis becomes a large part of the cure. Clearly defining the problem helps focus the patient and the practitioner on the resources necessary to reach an acceptable resolution.

Dealing with Multiple Problems

In the course of an interview, the practitioner often finds that the patient has multiple problems. Here, again, having a practical structure for dealing with these problems is helpful both in keeping the practitioner focused and meeting the patient's needs. If an unexpected emotional response occurs during the interview, the practitioner finds out what is going on, explores the issue with the three questions, "How does that make you feel?" "What troubles you the most?" and "How can you handle that?" then effects closure with an empathic statement. In this way, a simple technique, sequentially applied, can effectively be used to handle complex situations. The following case, reported by one of our senior physicians in training, illustrates the principles we are promoting:

A new patient, a 38-year-old woman, presented with multiple concerns, including vaginal itching, dyspareunia, need for contraception, and frequent headaches. On further questioning, she was a working mother of three teenage children, widowed six years previously, and remarried one year ago. Family history was positive for hypertension and diabetes in her grandparents and multiple sclerosis (MS) in her mother. The mother was currently 56 years old and had been in a nursing home for 12 years. At this point in the interview, the patient appeared tearful but attempted to suppress the tears. I asked her what was going on and then used the rest of the BATHE technique. The patient started to cry, saying that she had not cried for years about her mother. I asked her what her mom had been like. She stated she had always admired her mother's energy and unselfishness, which was why she felt so guilty about having her in the nursing home. I empathized, and we went on. Subsequently, I found out that her mother's diagnosis had been made at the age of 38. I asked her what she thought might be causing her headaches. She said I shouldn't think she was crazy, but she had considered whether it might not be MS. I supported her by telling her that that was a natural concern under the circumstances and that I would do a thorough evaluation in that regard.

At this point, about 10 minutes into the interview, I pointed out that she had come with quite a few concerns and asked her which one she wanted most to deal with in this visit. She stated that she was most concerned about her vaginal itch. After some routine questions regarding the genitourinary (GU) system, I asked how this condition was affecting her sexuality, to which she replied that she and her husband had not slept together in six months! She stated that she suspected him of having an affair. Six months ago also corresponded to the anniversary of her first husband's death. I asked a background question about the circumstances of her marriage and again finished the BATHE sequence. I then asked her to prepare for the physical examination and assured her I would check for venereal disease. She appeared relieved and revealed that she had also had a "fling" just before the onset of the itching.

During the physical exam, I did enough of a review of systems to assure myself that her headaches were not of an immediately serious nature, and I reassured her regarding her pelvic exam. I supported her by stating that she seemed to be handling things well under such stressful circumstances. I asked her to make an appointment for evaluation of her headaches and further discussion of her other concerns, including contraception. I asked her if she had any questions, and she said no but that she was very relieved after talking with me. The entire session lasted 25 minutes.

In this case, the practitioner sequentially dealt with a variety of problems, related to both present circumstances and unresolved grief from the past. By repeatedly using the BATHE structure, she dealt with these problems in a timely, effective, and sensitive manner.

The Resistant Patient

Certainly there are patients who are highly invested in separating their physical symptoms from their emotional states. Somatization is commonly seen in primary care across cultures and is generally associated with significant health problems and disabilities.[17] A few patients may be taken aback when questioned by their practitioners about what is going on in their lives. They may respond with "nothing." The practitioner has several choices when this happens. First, the subject can be dropped. We do not recommend this, because it reinforces somatization and wastes an opportunity to help the patient learn to connect physical conditions to emotional states. The second option, to repeat the word "nothing" with a questioning inflection, often results in the patient hesitantly revealing some current problem or a list of chronic annoyances. The rest of the BATHE sequence is then followed. The third option is simply to continue with the BATHE protocol, asking how the patient feels about the fact that nothing is going on. Practitioners tell us that they get some fascinating responses, such as the following common examples: "Just dreadful. I'm bored to tears." "Kind of mad, I guess. I'm tired of the same old thing!" "Awful. By now I was expecting to be promoted and nothing has happened." Regardless of the patient's reaction, BATHE usually provides important insights for the patient, as the following case illustrates:

A 29-year-old woman came to the Family Practice Center complaining of having had a headache for four days. Her past history included headaches that started 12 years previously and recurred intermittently around the time of her period. After getting a complete description of her symptoms and the history of the present illness, the young physician in training, who was not the patient's regular doctor, asked her what was going on in her life. She replied, "Nothing." "How do you feel about that?" he continued as taught. "How am I supposed to feel with nothing going on?" He tried one more time. "What about it troubles you the most?" She seemed exasperated, "What is supposed to trouble me when there is nothing going on in my life?" The doctor dropped the subject and proceeded with his exam.

Discussion of the case with the preceptor led to the conclusion that, in spite of the patient's denial, this was most likely a muscle tension headache, probably precipitated by stress or conflict. A decision was made to treat. When the doctor went back into the examination room and gave the patient her prescription for an analgesic, he gently posited, "There is something going on in your life, isn't there? You just don't want to talk with me about it."

The patient looked at him with admiration and smiled slightly. He suggested that she might want to come back and talk with her regular doctor. The clinician felt terrific. There had been a moment of real communication. He was sure that the patient had felt it also.

Patients Report They Like Being BATHEd

Some medical students, doctors in graduate training, practicing physicians, physicians' assistants and nurse practitioners attending our workshops have expressed concerns that the BATHE questions might not always be an appropriate addition to a medical history. They were afraid that patients might feel that the practitioner was being invasive of patients' personal space, asking for irrelevant information and might even offend patients. As in the case just described, of course, there are times when a particular patient may feel uncomfortable discussing personal issues, but in general our experience has been that patients are delighted to have the practitioner express interest in what is significant in their lives and that the technique helps to establish rapport. Until lately, we had only anecdotal evidence to support this view. Now a study by Leiblum and her colleagues[3] has found that use of the BATHE technique significantly increased patients' overall satisfaction with their outpatient visits. These researchers used an assistant to recruit and randomize 80 patients in the waiting room of a Family Practice Center, and to instruct four experienced physicians to either BATHE ten consecutive patients or provide usual care. The research assistant collected data from the patients after the visit. Outcome measures were based on the Healthcare Effectiveness Data and Information Set (HEDIS)[18] measures of patient satisfaction as interpreted by Press Ganey[19] Scores, widely used by organizations in the United States that evaluate physician practices. BATHEd patients reported significantly more positive impressions of doctors' concern, explanations of problems, efforts to include the patient in decision making, information about medications, instructions about follow-up care, amount of time spent, likelihood of recommending the physician to others and overall satisfaction with that particular visit.[3]

WHEN THE PATIENT COMES BACK TO TALK

Subsequent chapters will provide many specific suggestions and techniques for use in a 15-minute visit. At this point, let us look briefly at how Dr. Alan Buchanan, a psychiatrist at the University of British Columbia, has used the BATHE protocol to teach primary care physicians how to structure a 10-minute "counseling session."[20]

B stands for background. The opening two minutes belong to the patient. You open with "Tell me what's been going on since our last visit." The underlying message is that the practitioner is **there** to listen to the patient – and there is no need to rush.

A stands for affect (the feeling state). Summarize the feelings. The underlying message is "I have been listening." Dr. Buchanan suggests that since many patients cannot label feelings on their own, this can be very helpful to them.

T stands for trouble. "What is the worst thing about this situation?" The underlying message is a combination of "we can talk about anything here" and "our time is short so we must focus."

H stands for handling. "And how did you handle this?" sends the message that "you can handle this situation." What is important here is to manage this crisis, not to get stuck in overwhelming feelings.

E stands for empathy. Normalize the patient's reaction to the crisis. "It sounds awful, and I agree with what you have done so far – anybody would have had problems with this situation."

In the final few minutes, the physician asks, "What is the best thing that has happened lately?" Dr. Buchanan comments that this sometimes injects humor or initiates the process of seeing the crisis as an opportunity for change. Then the physician states, "For the next time I'd like you to (write the problem out in detail, or write down some options available, or reach out to some specific sources of support)." The underlying message is "You *can* handle this situation."

He ends the interview with a closing statement: "I'm glad we had a chance to talk about this," "I feel like I know you better," or just, "Sorry, but our time is up for today."

In later chapters more will be said about how to structure visits when the patient comes back to talk as well as the importance of focusing on something positive in the patient's life.

THE USE OF MEDICATION

One of the beauties of providing psychotherapeutic intervention in primary care is the option to combine talk therapy with medication. The individual practitioner must determine how and when to prescribe pharmacological treatment to ease the patient's symptoms. In general, when you screen for anxiety or depression by using the BATHE technique and determine that the patients' acute distress is so severe as to seriously interfere with their functioning, you may want to use medication to alleviate their symptoms. When patients are not able to sleep it is difficult to restore some measure of equilibrium. In treating depression, the practitioner has the option of prescribing psychotropic medication along with providing supportive therapy. Unfortunately, studies show that doctors do not necessarily talk with patients often once a diagnosis is made and a prescription issued.[21] It is critical to help patients develop realistic expectations about the action of the medication as well as to help them to handle the problematic aspects of their current situations.

Although medication can be extremely useful in managing acute problems, treating symptoms without addressing the underlying causes of a chronic problem perpetuates a patient's sense of powerlessness and hopelessness. A prescription for alprazolam (Xanax) does nothing to fix a bad marriage where communications have broken down. Patients need to be mobilized to change their behavior. If the patient is requesting medication, however, this provides an opportunity to bond with the patient. Later, an ongoing negotiation may be required to taper the medication over time.

BATHE: A USEFUL TECHNIQUE FOR MANY REASONS

As discussed earlier, the BATHE technique was originally designed to help practitioners determine the psychosocial background underlying the biomedical problems presented by patients, to establish rapport with patients and to serve as a rough screening test for anxiety, depression and situational stress disorders. Ideally, the questions will be posed in the order presented after the history of present illness has been elicited. We promote using the questions in the order presented, but also encourage use of the individual questions during other parts of the interview, when it seems appropriate to ask how something made the patient feel, what troubled them the most, or how they handled something. Statements of empathy are always encouraged when patients reveal some traumatic material.

Over the years, clinicians have discovered many other indications for the use of the BATHE technique. For example: When breaking bad news, to explore a patient's reaction to a diagnosis; to address lack of adherence to prescribed treatment, requests for inappropriate referrals or other difficult situations in the doctor/patient relationship. BATHE can be used to explore barriers to making positive life-style changes. It can be used to handle an unexpected revelation at the end of an interview or to probe for psychosocial precipitants related to somatic complaints; finally, BATHE can be used to educate patients regarding the interaction between their bodies and their minds.

Differentiating Approaches for Chronic and Acute Problems

The BATHE technique is useful for determining whether a problem is chronic or acute. Different approaches depend on this classification.[22] There are different underlying stories that must be considered.

Treating Acute Conditions

The medical model lends itself quite well to dealing with acute situations and/ or very dependent patients. The underlying story in acute situations is that the patient is not to blame for creating the problem – the patient is sick. The practitioner therefore takes responsibility for finding a solution for the problem: to diagnose, counsel, suggest, prescribe, and give orders that must be followed. All that is required of the patient is to comply with the treatment. This helps the patient to feel secure. The more acute the problem, the more important it is for the practitioner to take charge, at least temporarily. The practitioner makes suggestions and guides the patient in handling the situation. Close follow-up is necessary so that the patient feels supported and connected. In an emergency situation, and emergency for the patient is a subjective state, authoritarian behavior relieves anxiety. Ultimately, however, responsibility and control need to be returned to the patient.

Managing Chronic Problems

When dealing with chronic problems a useful approach also employs the story that patients are not to blame for creating their problems. They may have been abused, uninformed, or otherwise deprived. Perhaps it was circumstance, karma, bad parenting, some unavoidable breakdown, inexperience, or just bad judgment. Regardless, this story says that the patient is responsible for effecting solutions. The patient may begin by asking for and accepting help, coping constructively with the problem, and using it as a learning opportunity. In dealing with patients who are having chronic problems, this is a very useful approach. The removal of blame for creation of the problem is therapeutic. It relieves guilt and raises the patient's level of self-esteem. Although no blame is placed for developing chronically difficult situations, the patient is expected to take responsibility for dealing with these problems constructively and finding solutions. The practitioner will help, be a sounding board, and lead the cheering section, but the patient retains responsibility for managing the problem. The practitioner's positive expectation regarding the patient's ability to resolve the problem – the infusion of hope – is a powerful therapeutic tool.

Actually, the practitioner may believe the patient to be responsible for creating the problem, as in the case of the 38-year-old woman who had had a "fling"; however, pointing this out is rarely therapeutic since it underscores the patient's sense of hopelessness, guilt, and self-deprecation. Relieving patients of blame allows them to direct their energies outward, to work on solving their problems or transforming their environments without wasting energy berating themselves for creating these problems or permitting others to create them.[15]

As we have seen, determining whether a problem is chronic or acute allows the practitioner to choose the more effective therapeutic strategy. In either case, BATHE maintains the focus on the problem and how the patient might deal with it. In general, empowering patients and holding them responsible for finding solutions fosters self-esteem. However, when patients are in crisis, the practitioner may want to take a more active role and satisfy dependency needs. In either case, the patient feels better and functions better.

Engaging the Patient in a Psychotherapeutic Contract

After the physical examination and medical management decisions have been made, the practitioner returns to the information elicited by the BATHE technique. Determining the nature of the problem and giving an empathic response constitute a psychotherapeutic intervention. As has been stated, it focuses the patient and legitimizes his or her feelings. The practitioner now suggests that regardless of the origin of the problem, little can be gained by placing blame. Rather, it is important to determine what can be done and to evaluate the available options to manage the situation. The practitioner becomes the patient's ally in dealing with the problem. One approach is to advise the patient to take some time to think about it and return in one or two weeks if the problem is not resolved. If a patient is feeling overwhelmed and problems are numerous and complex, a contract, specifically a verbal understanding, is made for follow-up. It is helpful to specify that the practitioner will meet with the patient for a particular number of sessions or to discuss referral.

In later chapters we will discuss specific considerations that must be applied to patients presenting with certain problems, or perhaps we should say certain problem patients: hypochondriacs, depressed, suicidal, or grieving patients. All these lend themselves to therapeutic intervention by the primary care practitioner, provided that the contract is made clear. The practitioner's role, commitment, and limitations must be clearly spelled out. The patient's responsibilities must also be stated, acknowledged, and documented in the chart. Once a patient recognizes the need for a therapeutic process, referral to a mental health professional providing collaborative care is a superb option. The BATHE technique enables practitioners to identify patients who need these services. Any time the practitioner feels overwhelmed by the extent of the patient's problems, a psychiatric consult or referral is indicated. Patients to be referred include psychotic, addicted, or violent patients or any patient whose condition makes the practitioner feel uncomfortable. When referring a patient, there is an understanding that the practitioner will continue to be involved with the patient and continue to provide ongoing medical care.

Example: the Grieving Patient

Patients are often overcome when they suffer significant losses. Traumatic grief has been shown to negatively affect both physical and psychological health.[23] When working with a bereaved patient, or discovering a situation of unresolved grief during a routine BATHE inquiry, the practitioner should explain the need for working through feelings related to significant relationships that have been terminated through death or other circumstances. Grief work can usually be accomplished in six or eight sessions.

The process of mourning requires that patients come to terms with both the positive and negative feelings related to the person who is gone. It requires the patient to reflect, remember, and process significant milestones in the relationship. Much of this work can be done by writing about the deceased person, their history, and characteristics.[24] Patients should also be encouraged to look at photographs, talk with friends and relatives, and regularly check in with the practitioner to report on their progress. Although this can be a painful process, it is necessary in order to bring closure and allow the survivor to reengage with life.

The practitioner may contract with the patient for six or eight sessions to supervise the grief work or can refer the patient to a collaborating mental health practitioner or an ongoing support group. In any case, therapy must focus on reviewing the significant aspects of the terminated relationship, accepting the pain and finality of the loss, coming to terms with the good and bad aspects, and finally letting go.

THE EFFICACY OF TIME

Using the framework of *The Fifteen Minute Hour*, the practitioner provides focused attention and a safe environment for the patient to tell and assess some aspect of his or her story. The patient is invited to reexamine responses to situations, look at options, chart new goals, and acquire a more positive sense of self-efficacy. The clinician provides a structure for the patient to examine one particular problem and suggests that the patient will be able to replicate the process.

The time constraint is useful because it prevents overloading the patient and adding to the confusion. The practitioner conveys optimism that problems can be resolved one at a time and indicates that he or she is there to help the patient work through the problems. By returning to patients the sense of having some potential for affecting the course of their lives, for making their own decisions and choices, the practitioner is acting in a most highly therapeutic manner. In addition, when the practitioner routinely incorporates BATHE into every patient encounter, efficiency is built into the practice. A little energy invested in this process on each visit fosters the image of the practitioner as an empathic and involved figure. As a result, the practitioner is able to handle the patient's problems in an effective and timely fashion often before they assume overwhelming proportions.

ONE LAST POINT

In addition to asking patients the right questions, it is important to make sure everyone involved in the patient encounter is listening. Your listening skills and also the patient's are vital to resolving medical problems and promoting healing.[25]

SUMMARY

Many benefits accrue from assessing a patient's emotional status as part of each visit. Every physical complaint or office visit should be seen in the context of the patient's and his or her family's total life situation. The therapeutic effect grows out of the practitioner-patient relationship. The letters "BATHE" represent an acronym to recall a framework for handling the context of the visit. "B" stands for background: "What is going on?" "A" stands for affect: "How do you feel about it?" "T" stands for trouble: "What about it bothers you most?" "H" stands for handling: "How are you dealing with that?" "E" stands for empathy: "That must be very difficult for you!"

BATHEing the patient early in the interview structures an effective and efficient psychotherapeutic intervention into every patient encounter. BATHE has been shown to improve patient satisfaction with a visit. Multiple problems can be handled by sequentially applying the simple technique. BATHE can also be used to structure a return visit and to determine whether a problem is chronic or acute. The practitioner may wish to use medication as an adjunct to talk therapy. In acute situations it is useful for practitioners to take an active role in finding solutions, whereas chronic problems require that patients be held responsible for problem resolution. Any time the practitioner feels overwhelmed by the extent of a patient's problems, a psychiatric consult or referral should be considered.

The time constraint inherent in the brief session is useful because it prevents overloading the patient. The practitioner's optimism and focus on one problem at a time are an effective strategy and provide a model for further work. Attentive listening is a prerequisite for positive outcomes.

References

1. McQuaid JR, Stein MB, Laffaye D, *et al.* Depression in a primary care clinic: The prevalence and impact of an unrecognized disorder. *J Affect Disord.* 1999; **55**: 1–10.
2. Stein MB. Attending to anxiety disorders in primary care. *J Clin Psychiatry.* 2003; **64**(Suppl. 15): 35–9.
3. Leiblum SL, Schnall E, Seehuus M, *et al.* To BATHE or not to BATHE: patient satisfaction with visits to their family medicine physician. *Fam Med.* 2008 **40**(6): 407–11.
4. Vaillant GE. *Adaptation to Life.* Boston: Little, Brown & Co.; 1977.
5. Weed LL. *Medical Records, Medical Education, and Patient Care.* Cleveland: The Press of Case Western Reserve; 1969.
6. Kallman H, Stuart MR. BATH – a simple mnemonic to integrate psychosocial data into a soaped chart. Unpublished manuscript, 1980.
7. Tallia AF. *Verbal communication.* 1981. (Suggested adding "E for "Empathy" to the mnemonic BATH to create the acronym BATHE.)
8. Serido J, Almeida DM, Wethington E. Chronic stressors and daily hassles: unique and interactive relationships with psychological distress. *J Health Soc Behav.* 2004; **45**(1): 17–33.
9. Stewart M, Brown JB, Weston WW, *et al. Patient-Centered Medicine: transforming the clinical method.* Thousand Oaks, CA: Sage Publications; 1995.

10. Barsky AJ, Orav EJ, Bates DW. Somatization increases medical utilization and costs independent of psychiatric and medical comorbidity. *Arch Gen Psychiatry*. 2005; **62**(8): 903–10.

11. Gureje O, Simon GE, Ustun TB, *et al.* Somatization in cross-cultural perspective: a World Health Organization study in primary care. *Am J Psychiatry*. 1997; **154**: 989–95.

12. Cameron LD, Leventhal H, Leventhal A. Symptom ambiguity, life stress, and decisions to seek medical care. *Psychosom Med*. 1995; **57**: 37–47.

13. Bertakis KD, Roter D, Putnam SM. The relationship of physician medical interview style to patient satisfaction. *J Fam Pract*. 1991; **32**(2): 175–81.

14. Roter D. The enduring and evolving nature of the patient-physician relationship. *Patient Educ Couns*. 2000; **39**(1): 5–15.

15. Glass TA, Matchar DB, Belyea M, *et al.* Impact of social support on outcome of first stroke. *Stroke*. 1993; **24**(1): 64–70.

16. House JS, Landis KR, Umberson D. Social relationships and health. *Science*. 1988; **241**: 540–5.

17. Epstein RM, Quill TE, McWhinney IR. Somatization reconsidered. *Arch Intern Med*. 1999; **159**(3): 215–22.

18. National Committee for Quality Assurance (NCQA). NCQA Quality Compass. Available at: web.ncqa.org/tabid/177/Default.aspx

19. Press Ganey Associates Inc. Available at: www.pressganey.com/cs/research_and_analysis/patient_satisfaction (accessed 28 February 2008).

20. Buchanan A. *Counseling tips for family practitioners*. In: Sehon A, Buchanan A. Vancouver, B.C.: Sehon-Buchanan Medical Media. p. 82.

21. Meredith L, Wells KB, Kaplan SH, *et al.* Counseling typically provided for depression. *Arch Gen Psychiatry*. 1996; **53**: 905–12.

22. Brickman P, Rabinowitz VC, Karuza J, *et al.* Models of helping and coping. *Am Psychol*. 1982; **37**: 368–84.

23. Prigerson HG, Bierhals AJ, Kasl SV, *et al.* Traumatic grief as a risk factor for mental and physical morbidity. *Am J Psychiatry*. 1997; **154**(5): 616–23.

24. Pennebaker JW. Putting stress into words: health, linguistic, and therapeutic implications. *Behav Res Ther*. 1993; **31**(6): 539–48.

25. Lieberman JA, Stuart MR, Robinson SA. Enhance the patient visit with counseling and listening skills. *Fam Pract Manag*. 1996; **3**(10): 70–5.

CHAPTER 5

Rationale and Techniques for Fifteen-Minute Therapy

Patients generally assume that their practitioners are technically competent to diagnose and treat disease. Expressing interest in the patient and demonstrating warmth and support, particularly in the presence of debilitating, painful, or frightening symptoms, is a therapeutic gift.

In one of his seminal writings McWhinney[1] pointed out that practitioners are much more adept at applying the biological and physical sciences to the practice of medicine than they are in utilizing knowledge from the behavioral sciences. Every patient with a biomedical illness also "exhibits some form of behavior." It is important that practitioners pay attention to this behavior, as well as to the social context of the patient's symptoms. Even when psychiatric symptoms are the chief complaint, McWhinney states that most of the emotional disorders in general medical practice fall into the category of "problems of living," that is, the natural anxiety of people who are responding to perceived threats to their health or well-being. We cannot agree more! Although a patient's response to illness is determined by many factors, including genetic makeup, early history, previous experience with illness, current life situation, and aspirations for the future, the reaction to the current life situation is probably the most amenable to modification by the practitioner. For this reason, it is critical for the practitioner to routinely ask all patients about what is going on in their lives.

ROUTINELY INQUIRING ABOUT CURRENT LIFE SITUATIONS

Since patients' presenting problems are usually a complex amalgamation of physical, psychological, and social factors, ascertaining the situational context of the patient's visit helps the practitioner understand the significance of the patient's symptomatology and evaluate its severity.

Sickness Is Often Triggered by Psychological or Social Stress

The list of psychological factors that may precipitate illness is extensive. McWhinney[1] devised a taxonomy that identified seven general areas:
1. loss: either personal, such as bereavement or divorce, or loss of something valued, such as a home, position, or object
2. conflict: interpersonal or intrapersonal, having to do with conflicting internal demands
3. change: either triggered by life cycle events or a geographical event
4. maladjustment: interpersonal problems not having to do with acute conflicts; failure to adjust to occupational or home demands
5. other stresses, acute or chronic
6. general isolation
7. failure or frustrated expectations.

We would add to this list:
8. any anniversary of a significant loss or traumatic event.[2-4]

These types of situations negatively impact the health of the patient. They are also the situations that lower the patient's threshold of tolerance for the discomfort of symptoms or the threshold for anxiety about symptoms. Since patients are often not aware of this relationship, they are very relieved when the practitioner helps them to make this connection. According to McWhinney,[5] sometimes the aim of therapy may not be to remove the symptoms but to help the patient to live with them.

Stress Often Exacerbates Chronic Conditions

A person whose diabetes has been well controlled for years may suddenly present in the office because of an increased blood sugar determined by home glucose monitoring. Perhaps the most important question that the practitioner can ask is "What is going on in your life?" It may turn out that the patient is afraid of getting fired, his wife is threatening to leave him, a teenage daughter has an older boyfriend who is making sexual demands on her, or perhaps there are financial problems related to college costs for children or increases in mortgage payments. These or any other situational stresses can easily precipitate an exacerbation of the diabetes and can best be managed with a psychological rather than a chemical intervention.

Diabetes is not the only chronic condition affected by stress. Consider the following case related by one of our colleagues:

> A 33-year-old female came to see me with a chief complaint of difficulty breathing. She reported a two-day history of shortness of breath, especially with exertion, and a need for increased use of her albuterol inhaler. Other than a history of mild to

moderate asthma, she has no significant medical problems. Her asthma occasionally flares up with seasonal changes, allergies, and strenuous exercise, but it is easily controlled with inhalers. She is married and has two young children. She works full-time outside the home. She reported no other symptoms, such as cough, sore throat, rhinorrhea, sneezing, fever, nausea, vomiting, or rash. Her allergies were well controlled with 10 mg of loratadine (Claritin) daily.

At this particular visit, the patient appeared fatigued and anxious. As I asked her questions about her breathing and other symptoms, she tried to minimize her disease and stated she just wanted renewals for her inhalers. At this point I decided to BATHE the patient. When asked what was happening in her life, she relaxed somewhat and offered a litany of stressful events that had occurred in the past several days culminating in a major screaming match with one of her children. When I asked how she felt about this situation, she replied, "And in the middle of it all, I just started wheezing!" She went on to say that she was feeling overwhelmed and that what troubled her most was that her asthma was slowing her down and preventing her from addressing her family's needs in a timely fashion. I provided empathy and then we discussed ways in which she could cope, which included changing her inhaler regimen, stress management techniques, time management, and enlisting the help of her husband. She left the office appearing more relaxed and breathing easier.

The Practitioner's Interest Is Supportive

The practitioner's interest in the patient as a person is demonstrated by the inquiry about the social context of his or her problem. In this way, the practitioner demonstrates warmth and caring and affirms the individuality and importance of the patient. The patient has to make sense out of the practitioner's show of interest. One explanation is that the practitioner is a warm and caring person. This makes the patient feel safe and in good hands. Another explanation is that the patient is a worthwhile person who has some significance for the practitioner. This also makes the patient feel good. In either case, the patient will feel supported and hence be able to tolerate symptoms better.[6]

When practitioners routinely inquire into the circumstances of a patient's life, the patient becomes aware of the physical-psychological interaction. Understanding the effects of stress on the physical responses of the body helps to make the patient feel more in control and therefore less anxious. Becoming aware of the effects of stress is a prerequisite for learning to manage it. One of our faculty members related the following case of a 36-year-old divorced social worker currently living with a "significant other":

F.L. presented with severe stomach cramps and wondered if she had ovarian cancer. A quick BATHE revealed high stress at work, which may also have accounted for her slightly low white blood cell count and elevated cholesterol. During the follow-up phone call to discuss the test results, the patient suddenly volunteered that she only gets the stomach cramps when there is high stress at work.

If we are not aware that we are becoming tense, there is no behavioral cue for applying relaxation techniques, be they physical or cognitive. Precipitants of stress are not always directly connected to the current situation. Understanding the significance of an anniversary, its potential for precipitating illness, and the high correlation of anniversaries with accidents[2,3] can keep patients from overreacting, turning acute events into chronic conditions, and setting unrealistic expectations for themselves.

A patient will almost sheepishly present with chest pain on the anniversary of his father's heart attack, saying, "I know it's probably psychosomatic, Doc, but check it out anyway and relieve my anxiety. Every year at this time, I seem to develop these symptoms." After ruling out the acute condition and reassuring the patient, it is appropriate to encourage the patient to reassess his relationship with his father. If he has not adequately dealt with his grief, it is important for him to focus on both the good and bad memories of his youth and come to terms with his remaining ambivalent feelings. This can be accomplished by writing about his father and their relationship, as will be discussed later.

Eliciting Patients' Reactions

Once the practitioner has determined the context of the visit in terms of what is going on in the patient's life, it is important to inquire about the patient's emotional reaction. "How do you feel about that?" is the most efficient question to ask, rather than "Why do you think this is happening?" or "What does your wife think about it?" The point is to get the patient to make an affective response. "How do you feel about it?" usually prompts a response that starts with "I feel . . .." If the patient starts to offer other information or starts with "I feel that" followed by a judgment, it is important that the practitioner interrupt and persist, "Yes, I understand, but how does it make you feel?" We have explained earlier that if you can substitute the word "think" for the word "feel," you are expressing an opinion rather than an emotion. "I feel that" always signals that the patient is making a judgment, rather than expressing a feeling. Additionally, we would caution practitioners not to get caught up in the details of the patient's situation. Finding out who said what to whom has no therapeutic significance. It is best to briefly summarize the situation and proceed to the next question.

Our goal for the patient is to label and express feelings, giving us the opportunity to empathize. Then we attempt to focus the patient on a problem-solving strategy. Often, patients may admit to feeling anxious or depressed. Just having the patient acknowledge, "I am angry," or "I am sad," or "I feel rejected," "scared," "powerless," "overwhelmed," or "totally confused" is therapeutic. Most people react automatically or semi-automatically to most of the events in their lives without any conscious awareness or thought about what they are feeling. When we focus their attention on their current affective experience, we break that pattern. When feelings are experienced, accepted, and acknowledged, they do not need to become psychosomatic symptoms. This is the essence of an effective psychotherapeutic intervention.

Teaching a Process

When the practitioner inquires about how the patient is feeling about a specific situation, the focus changes from what is happening to how the patient is reacting. This models a process that puts the emphasis on the patient's reactions while demonstrating the practitioner's concern. The clinician extends an invitation to get at the root of what is actually troubling the patient. Some patients have extreme difficulty in identifying or labeling their feelings. Their stories will focus on what happened and what they did or other people did in response. In this case the practitioner can use active listening as a way to focus on the affective domain: "Sounds like you were surprised and hurt when your request was denied. Or were you angry?" This gives the patient the opportunity to reflect on the feelings that might have been experienced. Finally, it is important to follow up by asking "What about it troubled you the most?"

By inquiring about the significance of the event, the practitioner in a subtle way implies that the interpretation about what is troubling the patient is not necessarily obvious. This simple device may prepare the patient to see the situation as less catastrophic than had been assumed. It may also help the patient to recognize the need to develop potential solutions. The practitioner implies no meaning or judgment. The same situation has different significance for different people. The nonjudgmental nature of the practitioner's response makes the patient feel accepted and creates the conditions necessary to promote psychological change.[7]

As part of the initial inquiry, the practitioner now has a choice. One option is to ask the patient how the situation is being handled and then make an empathic response. The other option is to first acknowledge that the situation must be difficult and then to ask how the patient might handle it.

Many practitioners schedule patients with emotional problems for the end of the day in order to leave time to explore the situation fully. We strongly recommend against this practice, since it involves too much of an investment of valuable time on the part of the practitioner, creates unrealistic expectations on the part of the patient, and may not necessarily result in increased therapeutic benefits. Given a positive doctor-patient relationship, little difference in outcome has been found among psychotherapeutic techniques.[8–10] We therefore strongly urge primary care practitioners to practice, over-learn (do them so often that they become automatic), and routinely use our techniques because they work and do not take much of the practitioner's time.

EDITING THE STORY

In Chapter 3 we defined psychotherapy as helping patients to edit their stories. It is clear that the stories we tell ourselves about who we are and of what we are capable determine how we will function in the world and to what extent we will achieve our potential. In other words, the stories we generate create our reality. This view is based on the postmodern understanding that we interpret our experienced reality through a pair of conceptual glasses – glasses based on factors such as our personal goals, our past experiences, our values and attitudes, our body of knowledge, the nature of the language we use, and our contemporary culture.[11] There is actually no way to observe the world as it really is with pure objectivity. This concept is very useful from a pragmatic therapeutic perspective. When we get the patient to consider a new story, we help him or her to create a new reality.

The Story Must Be Heard and Reflected Back with Empathy

Patients must be allowed to tell their stories. In order to make therapeutic interventions, we must first hear the patient's experience of pain, frustration, anxieties, and perceived limits. It is hoped that we can encourage patients to give us a brief synopsis rather than a multivolume saga. That is one of the functions of the BATHE technique. We cannot provide reassurance or remove impediments to adherence until we understand the patient's concerns. Using active listening by reflecting back the content of patients' concerns lets patients know that they have been heard and understood. When this is followed by empathic responses, patients feel competent as well as connected to the practitioner. This creates a highly therapeutic condition.

Challenging Limits

As was pointed out in Chapter 3, it is important to listen for the defining limits in the patient's narrative: the *always's, nevers, everyones, no ones,* and *can'ts.* These words help to define the patient as helpless. Filters that selectively process experience must be exposed before behavior can be changed. Absolutes must be challenged. This is also one of the major techniques of Cognitive Behavioral Therapy (CBT). One or two questions can help to clarify the situation: "You *always* make mistakes? You mean, you have *never* gotten anything right?" "*Everyone* is smarter than you?" "How many people have you tested?" "*No one* has ever supported you?" An appropriate response might be "I'm sorry, that must feel awful." (Translation: I support you.)

However, the most important intervention is in response to the phrase "I can't," a clue regarding a limited sense of self-efficacy. Given motivation, there are very few things that humans cannot accomplish. In every case, when patients complain that they cannot do something, the practitioner can respond with, "You have not been able to do that until now."

The Amazing Power of the Word "yet"

The word "yet" implies that something is about to happen or will happen in the future. It also implies that it is possible. When patients state that they cannot do something, they are basing that assertion on past experience. When practitioners respond that patients have not been able to do it "yet," the implication is that the practitioner expects the patient to be able to accomplish whatever it is in the future. That is a powerful suggestion coming from a highly influential person. It challenges the patient's story and promotes change. It is important for the practitioner to make the statement with assurance (it is always true). Other phrases, such as "Up to now this has been difficult for you" or "Up until this time you haven't succeeded at this," are equally useful; but we like the word "yet." It is short and to the point, and when you use it: *Y*ou *E*mpower *T*hem.

Listening for limits highlighted by patients' statements about what they cannot do and responding with a counter statement that they "just haven't yet" constitutes a very practical therapeutic intervention. When the patient returns for the next visit it is likely that he or she will state that whatever it was has not been accomplished *yet*, but . . .. The practitioner will know that the message has been heard and is being processed. Change will follow. The patient's story is being edited.

Aiming for Small Wins

We have previously pointed out that it is the feeling of powerlessness, or of demoralization, that brings a patient to a therapist.[12] It is feeling helpless in the face of threat that is devastating, physically and mentally.[13] In many cases, the overwhelming scope of problems faced by individuals, and for that matter, by society as a whole, predisposes people to feeling helpless, since there appears to be little that can be done to effect any kind of meaning-ful solution. According to K.E. Weick,[14] attempted large-scale solutions to overwhelming societal problems, such as crime, traffic congestion, and pollution, and we might add terrorism, often create new problems, such as the need for increased law enforcement and security removing needed funds from other services; multilane highways drawing more people away from public transportation, and the cost of pollution control, raising taxes. The most detrimental aspect of the situation, however, is that people's level of arousal gets raised without them having access to responses that will effectively impact the situation. This is the essence of *stress*. People go on allostatic overload because they perceive the severity and intensity of the problem while feeling totally helpless to do anything about it.

The corrective strategy proposed by Weick[14] is to focus on minor leverage points that enable people to engage in productive problem solving. In other words, people can act to make other people aware of the problem, organize rallies, write letters, wear red, white and blue ribbons, get attention from the newspapers, reuse and recycle and in that way feel as though they are accomplishing something. They are not just standing idly by, watching the world go to ruin.

Achieving small wins has the effect of reversing both the over-arousal and apathy that result from feeling demoralized. Focusing patients on small wins provides practical, immediate, and surprisingly effective results since it lowers their levels of psychological distress, that is, gets them off *tilt*. This is a therapeutic milestone. Getting patients to focus on a minor change in their own behavior – slightly changing a schedule, carving out time for themselves, organizing a list, clearly asking for something they want, calling a friend, expressing feelings without attacking or blaming, writing a letter, or even sending a postcard – can result in a small win. Successfully doing one little task provides a sense of having some power, and there is less risk for patients when they tackle a problem in stages, since less is riding on each particular behavior. Not only is the outcome more likely to be positive, but also it will be less traumatic if it is not. The main idea is to make patients aware that their actions can make a difference. Weick explained as follows:

> Brief therapy is most successful when the client (patient) is persuaded to do just one thing differently that interdicts the pattern of attempted solutions up to that point. Extremely easy or extremely difficult goals are less compelling than are goals set closer to perceived capabilities. Learning tends to occur in small increments rather than in an all-or-none fashion.[15]

Small wins increase the chance of success, foster optimism, help people to refocus their energy productively, and restore belief in personal control. The effectiveness of the intervention grows out of the practitioner's faith in the patient's ability to effect small, meaningful changes. This subject also has relevance for counseling patients to make lifestyle changes, as will be discussed later.

THE IMPORTANCE OF STRUCTURE

Ordinarily, when a practitioner invites a patient to talk without structuring the interview, it is possible that the patient will gain some benefit, but it can be a process that is quite random. In our experience patients will complain incessantly and repeatedly about the behavior of other people and circumstances that cannot be changed, thereby reinforcing their limited interpretations of their reality. Allowing patients to go on and on about these matters is counter-therapeutic. It tries the patience of the practitioner and sets up unreasonable expectations, on the part of the patient, regarding the amount of time the practitioner has available. Also, we often find that the longer the patient talks, the more upset he or she gets. When recalling a litany of insults and injuries experienced, patients rekindle many negative feelings. By giving the patient valuable time and listening attentively to unchanging complaints, the practitioner supports the patient's distorted perceptions and the story remains unchanged. Ultimately, the practitioner may decide that it is not worth trying to treat the psychological aspects of a patient's problems.

Perhaps, over time, the uncritical attention of the practitioner may enhance the patient's self-esteem. This is the major assumption behind Rogers's client-centered therapy.[7] However, in terms of time and energy invested, rather than letting patients continue to retell the same story, the more effective and economical strategy is to briefly summarize, give an empathic response, and then make one or two interventions that challenge or potentially change patients' behavior or assumptive world view, as in the following example:

A 55-year-old woman comes to the office complaining of fatigue. She says that she has been tired for weeks. She has had no physical exam for years. There is no significant medical history. Asked about what is going on in her life, she says that both she and her husband work full-time, she is also a homemaker, and she takes care of her 17-year-old son, who is legally blind but has just been accepted into college. She looks frightened, depressed, and essentially closed. Asked how she feels about what is going on, she only volunteers that she is tired. The physical exam is unremarkable; blood and urine tests and a pelvic exam all are normal. The practitioner asks, "Do you think that you might be depressed?" The patient replies, "Depressed? I don't know if I'm depressed. I know I'm tired. I work a 40-hour week. Keep my own house. Cook dinner every night. I have a nice husband who would be happy with a bologna sandwich but wouldn't make it for himself." She pauses and then says, "Oh yes, my sister cares for our 90-year-old father. I go over there every Saturday to help out. I really wish she'd put him in a nursing home, but I feel guilty when I think that, and my sister won't hear of it."

The practitioner (challenging the view that wishing to put the father into a nursing home is any cause for feeling guilty) responds that he thinks that that is a perfectly reasonable way to feel. The patient sighs. She looks relieved and volunteers that she has done nothing for herself in recent times. The practitioner suggests that she make just one small change. The patient smiles, "I can do that. Thank you so much, Doctor, I feel so much better."

As we have said previously, the therapeutic intervention consists of interrupting fixed patterns of behavior and thought by focusing attention either on the behavior or away from it (distracting the person and/or focusing on other options). By BATHEing the patient, we are focusing on feelings, on interpretations, and on the behavioral responses of the patient and setting the stage for change.

Frequently the initial sequence is all that is required in the way of psychological support. It often helps the patient to gain insight into the particular situation and make a plan for resolution. It is only with those patients whose situational stress is currently unmanageable that one needs to engage in a specific therapeutic contract.

Determining Number of Sessions

We know from crisis theory, as described by Gerald Caplan,[16] that an intense crisis situation is usually resolved in six to eight weeks. As discussed in Chapter 2, crisis is a time of major stress as people try to adapt to large-scale acute or anticipated change. During a period of crisis, patients tend to function much less efficiently than they normally do. People under stress regress to more primitive modes of behavior, have a narrower view, have a harder time with problem solving, and are not able see potential options. The practitioner's expressed support engages the patient's sense of well-being and provides an ally to help with the problem. In making a contract for follow-up, the practitioner commits to following the patient through the time of greatest stress. From crisis theory, it is obvious that six or eight weeks provide a reasonable expectation of problem resolution. The practitioner arranges to see the patient for brief sessions regularly during that time. Seeing the patient once each week is appropriate if the problem is serious. Once every other week is sufficient if the patient is less overwhelmed. If the patient is feeling totally unstrung, a twice-weekly contact may be necessary during the acute phase of the crisis.

By agreeing to see the patient regularly and briefly for a specified number of sessions, a message is conveyed that the problem is solvable and that the practitioner expects resolution to come within a reasonable period of time. Conveying this message is part of the therapeutic intervention. Hope is engaged since patients recognize that the practitioner is seeing factors that mitigate their feelings of despair. Perhaps the problem is manageable after all. Patients regain a sense of worth based on the practitioner wanting to engage with them to resolve the situation. It is a consistent message. Not only is the practitioner saying that the patient is worthy and deserving, but also the practitioner is making a commitment to work with the patient. The patient feels both more competent and connected. The fact that the practitioner places no blame but suggests that the problem needs to be resolved is practical.

Fielding Unexpected Reactions During the Interview

Often as part of taking a history, a routine question about previous hospitalizations, family illness, or previous geographical moves may elicit a strong emotional reaction in a patient, that is, trigger painful memories. The practitioner may be at a loss whether to ignore, soothe, or deeply explore the reaction. BATHEing provides a constructive alternative:

A young woman presented in the office complaining of a sore throat. Initial inquiry was unremarkable. However, when asked if there was any family history of rheumatic fever, she suddenly started to cry and recalled that while she was in high school she had been put to bed for several months because of rheumatic fever. The practitioner was first taken aback and hesitant to get into an old painful experience. However, since something had to be done, the doctor decided to apply the BATHE technique. She opened by inquiring about the background, "You were in high school, about what grade?"

"I was just starting my senior year."

Going right to affect, the physician asked, "And they put you on complete bed rest, how did you feel about that?"

The patient replied, "I felt so isolated and out of it."

The physician did not allow herself to explore these feelings further but inquired directly about trouble, "What about the situation troubled you the most?"

"I was afraid that I would not graduate with my class."

"How did you handle that?" was the final question.

"Well, there wasn't much I could do. I had to go to summer school. It was awful."

The empathic response followed, "I can see that that was a very difficult time for you. Tell me, any other serious illnesses?"

The patient responded, "No." Then after a pause, "You know, at this point it really doesn't make any difference. As a matter of fact, now that I think of it, I think I did better in college because I worked for a year first."

The physician responded, "I'm glad. Now I'd like to examine you and make sure that everything else is O.K."

VALUABLE STRATEGIES FOR EMPOWERING PATIENTS

Over the years we have found many effective interventions that can be used alone or in combination during a regular medical visit to change patients' perception of their ability to manage the problems in their lives. None take more than a minute or two to execute.

Helping the Patient to Explore Options

In dealing with a patient's situational stress, it is crucial that the practitioner not take responsibility for solving the patients' problems. In *The House of God*,[17] a biting satire about medical education, one of the primary truths (rule four) clearly states, "The patient is the one with the disease." If the patient is the one with the disease or the problem, the patient has a right to decide what, if anything, should be done about it. The practitioner has the opportunity to intervene in the process, first by making the patient aware that there are options and then by encouraging the patient to make a conscious choice about what to do. There are three useful strategies that can be presented to a patient: looking at the consequences, applying tincture of time, and choosing not to choose.

Looking at Consequences

The practitioner can encourage the patient to think about and/or list several possible courses of behavior and to sort out the consequences inherent in these choices. A good structure is to ask the patient to specify what the best and worst possible outcomes might be. Patients who are very angry often talk about wanting to kill the offending party. Rather than responding, "You don't mean that!" (Yes, they do, at least for the moment.) Or, "You can't do that!" (Yes, they can! It is not a good idea, but it is possible and unfortunately happens every day), the effective reply is "I can understand that you would feel that way, but that does not sound like a very practical option when you consider the consequences. Do you agree? O.K. Let's talk again next week after you think about what you might do that's more practical." The implication here is that the feeling is legitimate (It is!) but that once the patient thinks about it, other behavioral choices will appear. Also it is clear that the decision about what to do can be deferred at least until the following week. This relieves some pressure. The notion of "What is the worst thing that can happen if you do this?" is a very important one for the patient to explore. If the potential outcome is totally unacceptable, unless the probability of its occurring is definitely zero, the patient is advised not to consider that particular choice. These pragmatic instructions will help empower patients to view their circumstances more constructively.

Applying Tincture of Time

It is often true that the more important a decision is, the less information we have to base it on and the less time we take to make it. We put a deposit on a desirable house after one or two brief visits because if we do not act immediately, someone else will snap it up. Then we spend days choosing among shades of paint or wallpaper patterns.

Often a patient who is reacting emotionally to an event may feel impelled to make a decision. Having learned of her husband's unfaithfulness, a wife may feel she must either leave him immediately or have an affair herself. Neither of these options is likely to have a positive outcome. Instead, the practitioner encourages the patient to take time to sort out her feelings. Reacting to an acute loss involves an increased intensity of pain. This pain must be accepted and experienced fully. Ultimately it will lead to understanding and personal growth. The practitioner offers support and schedules an appointment to talk again. The implication is that tincture of time will provide relief.

Choosing not to choose

In a case where all apparent choices are unacceptable and the patient does not want to pick the lesser of the evils, the practitioner can instruct the patient that for the moment at least the best course of action may be to do nothing. Sometimes all the important information is not available to make an intelligent choice. The critical question to answer is now "What is the worst thing that can happen if you don't make a decision about this?" To choose not to choose is an option that many people never consider.

As we have said, psychological pain is something that must be felt but does not necessarily require a behavioral response. Often there is no need to act, especially if the pain is induced by the actions of another person over whom we have no control. In many cases, breaking a pattern by not acting in response to provocation by another shifts the balance of power. When I refuse to accept the conditions of a current relationship, it becomes the other person's problem to decide what to do. There are times that being "passive aggressive" really pays off. In general, when faced with several unacceptable choices, it is a good idea to make oneself comfortable while waiting for something to happen. It usually does.

Exploring Symbolic Meaning

One of the more fascinating aspects of practicing primary care medicine is the opportunity to engage meaningfully with a variety of people. The specialist who treats limited organ systems is only excited by unusual manifestations of disease and the opportunity to diagnose rare cases. The primary care practitioner can be endlessly fascinated by the varied reactions that different individuals have to the same circumstances. It is the particular meaning that each of us attributes to an event (the story) that determines our reaction, rather than the event itself. In every case where a person appears to be overreacting to a particular situation, we can assume that a symbolic meaning to that circumstance is triggering the patient's response, as shown by the following example:

Mr. Harris, a 28-year-old white male, presented in the emergency room with chest pain and difficulty breathing of sudden onset. He had no risk factors for heart disease, and examination, electrocardiogram, and enzyme studies were totally normal. The practitioner was aware that Mrs. Harris was due to deliver their first child momentarily and that the couple was extremely happy about the prospect of becoming parents. Arrangements were complete, and Mr. Harris had planned to stay with his wife during the delivery.

After reassuring the patient about the condition of his heart, the doctor inquired about what was currently happening. She was informed that the obstetrician had just told the couple that the baby was in breech position and that he had decided to do a cesarean delivery. At this point the patient started to cry. He revealed that he himself had been a breech delivery and that his mother had died in childbirth. He was sure that his wife would not survive. He had so wanted to be present at the birth but now could not face the prospect.

The practitioner was able to reassure him about the improvement in obstetrical procedures over the past 28 years and the relatively low risk associated with breech presentation when the baby is delivered by cesarean section. However, the physician did point out that it was perfectly O.K. to be concerned and scared. The patient was then able to connect his severe reaction to his own tragic birth circumstances rather than the current situation. The physician suggested that perhaps the patient needed to bring a support person to the hospital for himself. The following week, a proud father, gowned and masked, held his wife's hand in the operating room and watched his son take his first breath.

When helping a patient tie a particular reaction to its historical roots, the practitioner implies that the patient can break the pattern of response and reassess the significance of that situation in the present. Up to now, you may have a particular intolerance to people's loud arguing because when you were a child your parents fought bitterly. Listening to them, you felt helpless and frightened because your security was threatened. Whenever you heard people arguing, you felt helpless and frightened just as you did then. If a practitioner were to ask you gently, "Are you really helpless now? As an adult, is your security threatened when someone is shouting?", you would become aware of the change in your circumstances and learn to modify your reaction to loud arguments and, thereby, affect a change.

The practitioner's brief inquiry about the historical roots of an event can have a profound effect on a patient's self-esteem, sense of control, feelings of self-efficacy, and assumptive world view. It is not necessary to explore the circumstances, distortions, or details in depth. It is only necessary to point out to the patient that there appears to be an inconsistency in the severity of the reaction in relation to the apparent face value of the event. Once patients are in touch with the original onset of the problem they can be asked to write an autobiography, keep a journal of current reactions, or compare memories with various living relatives in order to sort out the origins of some of their stories and troubling interpersonal reactions. Often this will promote constructive dialogue between patients and the significant persons in their lives. The important issue is that the patient is the one who must understand and ultimately change the reaction. The practitioner's view of the situation, regardless how accurate, accomplishes nothing. As Shem has said, "The patient is the one with the disease."[17] The patient also is the one who must make the connections and change the responses.

Focusing the Patient in the Present

All reactions to current life stress are significantly affected by past experience. However, when engaging a patient in a brief therapy session, it is crucial to stress that regardless of a problem's origin or historical significance (fascinating as that may be), the past is past, and all we have to deal with is the present. Dwelling on past hurts is not useful: "Do you still resent your brother now, because your mother always favored him when you were kids? Really?" "Gee, I guess I do." "My guess is that your mother did the very best that she could. What would it take for you to forgive her?" The reality is that when we hold on to our grudges or nurse our resentments, our bodies pay a price.[18,19] We make ourselves miserable and do not actually affect the people with whom we are angry. In the past several years the interest in the effects of forgiveness has grown exponentially.[20,21] It is a process that can be taught, as discussed in Chapter 8.

Just as there is no benefit to obsessing about past hurts, assumptions made about the future are usually wrong and destructive. When a patient generalizes from a current unfavorable situation to speculate about a bleak outlook, the practitioner needs to challenge this distortion; for example, "I understand that your husband has left you and that you feel very hurt. However, it is not legitimate to assume that no one will ever love you again." "Yes, it is very painful to have your article rejected by the *AAI Journal.* You worked very hard on it and were sure it would be accepted. However, that does not mean that *no one* will ever publish it." "You are feeling very unhappy right now, but that does not mean that you will never be happy again." When a patient says, "I *know* that such and such will happen because it always has," it is important to correct him or her by restating, "You assume that such and such will happen. What is it that you could possibly do to change that?" Challenging the underlying irrational thinking, as we have pointed out previously, is an application of CBT.

It is important to encourage the patient to take one day at a time. If the patient is in extreme pain, it may be necessary to suggest taking it five minutes at a time. Then the patient is instructed to acknowledge that accomplishment. Patients should also be cautioned that wallowing in their pain is not constructive. If occasionally they cannot resist the need to wallow, they may be given permission to do so, providing they limit wallowing to five-minute sessions. Patients really respond quite well to this type of instruction. It puts their pain into context and gives them a sense of control.

These edicts, stated with the authority of the practitioner, and with the attributed social power inherent in the role, help the patient reassess the resources that are available for dealing with current problems. The practitioner's encouragement to appraise reality in the present, rather than dwelling on the past, which cannot be changed, or the future, which cannot be predicted accurately, is very productive. Patients are generally depressed about the past and anxious about the future. When we focus them in the present and engage them in constructive problem solving rather than fight or flight behavior, they respond amazingly well.

Three-step Problem Solving

We have promoted several "cookbook" approaches to therapy because they provide a simple structure through which to trigger a practitioner's efforts to help patients. In Chapter 3 we introduced the PLISSIT structure to determine levels of intervention from simple permission giving, to limited information, specific suggestions, and finally, a contract for intensive therapy. In Chapter 4, and the current chapter, we have repeatedly preached about the benefits of BATHEing the patient to determine and manage the situational context of the patient visit. Now we propose a three-step sequence of questions that can be effectively applied to any disturbing situation. These questions are as follows:

1. What am I feeling?
2. What do I want?
3. What can I do about it?

This is often a useful framework for practitioners to apply to their own reactions, as will be discussed in Chapter 9. For the present, let us focus back on the patient. The series of questions now becomes the following:

1. What are you feeling? (Label the actual feeling)
2. What do you want? (Specifically state your goal)
3. What can you do about it? (Focus on what you can control.)

For example, patient X is complaining about how his daughter's attitude disturbs him. The practitioner asks, "What are you feeling?" The patient may try to continue ranting about his daughter's behavior and give examples to illustrate that she is not acting the way she should be. He says they fight all the time and he screams at her. The practitioner persists, "What do you feel in that situation?" or "How do you *feel* about that?"

It may turn out that the patient feels angry, hurt, frightened, discounted, disappointed, devalued, disgusted, or some other unpleasant sensation depending on the meaning of his daughter's attitude for him.

At this point the practitioner acknowledges that feeling and asks, "What do you want?" At first the patient will respond that he does not want to be in this situation and he does not want his daughter to treat him this way. The practitioner persists, "What *do* you want?"

"I want her to change her behavior." (Sometimes patients say they do not really know, in which case the practitioner can encourage them to think about that and come back to talk again.)

The final question is "What can you do about that? I understand that fighting with her has not been helpful." The patient may decide that he can reward appropriate behavior, discuss it quietly, present the situation to his daughter as a problem to be solved, negotiate a contract, and let his daughter know that he truly loves and accepts her. Sometimes there is nothing that can be done. Once that becomes clear, what the patient feels about the situation changes to appropriate sadness. It is hard to accept the fact that we cannot control other people's attitudes and behavior.

In any case, this three-step process is a powerful therapeutic intervention because it labels feelings, clarifies what the patient wants, and points to a direction for achieving these goals. It is economical in time and direct in therapeutic value, since it encourages new ways of thinking and behaving while discouraging the passive role. It also teaches the patient a strategy that can be applied to any number of situations.

Putting the Patient Back in Control

We have said that the feeling of being overwhelmed is generally the trigger for patients' help-seeking behavior. When the practitioner engages the patient in problem solving, patients become aware that they have some control over the circumstances of their lives. Since the relationship with the practitioner is an ongoing one, patients sense that they have a partner and therefore feel less isolated. Someone cares and wants to follow their progress. If feelings of abandonment helped to trigger unpleasant reactions, now there is an assurance of ongoing support that will continue to be available over time. They feel connected.

The second important factor concerns patients' reactions to practitioners' expectations that they are capable of handling their situations. The practitioner clearly indicates to patients that their reactions are legitimate but that they have choices and that there are always actions available to them that will improve their current circumstances, if only slightly. If a patient is able to hear and accept these messages, it will change how the patient feels about his or her ability to cope. Certainly the patient is not helpless and will no longer feel hopeless. This change in reaction may even make the situation appear less difficult and ultimately improve it. Patients feel more competent. Consider the following case described by one of our graduates:

A 37-year-old, divorced, Egyptian female returned to the office for a follow-up visit for her elevated cholesterol and for her annual gynecologic exam. She appeared particularly sad today; she did not smile, and she spoke in a monotone voice. It was more difficult than usual to engage her in conversation. On review of systems, she had multiple somatic complaints, such as lower back pain, shoulder pain, and headaches. She also had several neurovegetative complaints: 12-pound weight gain over three to four months, lack of energy, fatigue, difficulty concentrating, and difficulty falling asleep. I was concerned that she was clinically depressed.

When I asked what was happening in her life at that time, she related that she felt a great deal of stress because of overwhelming responsibilities. She admitted that she worried too much and that she knew many of her symptoms might be related to her worries. She is a single mother of two teenage girls; she works full-time and attends school part-time at the local community college. When asked what troubled her the most, she admitted that her husband had deserted her and their children, leaving them here in the United States with her relatives, while he returned to Egypt with another woman and subsequently filed for divorce. She felt sad, angry, and bitter over these events.

When I asked how she was handling all this stress, she thought about it for a few seconds, and then her affect brightened as she replied that she normally maintains a positive outlook on life. She stated that her faith in God, and what He has in store for us, carries her through each difficult day. She also said that she is blessed to have multiple, strong family supports here in this country. The patient appeared quite relieved and justified when I empathized with her and pointed out that she was doing a great job holding herself and her family together, despite such adversity. The patient left the office smiling and thanking me for giving her permission to feel and express her emotions.

A constructive response to the practitioner's intervention will engage a positive cycle. We are all familiar with vicious cycles and downward spirals. Positive cycles are equally self-generating. When patients cease to feel overwhelmed, they resume their normal and more effective functioning. Mature coping mechanisms again become available. The patient's view of the situation broadens, and novel stimuli can be experienced and processed. This will lead to more effective problem solving and a better sense of being in control. This improved functioning will then be reinforced by success in achieving desired outcomes.

Focusing on Strengths

Every person or situation has both good and bad potential. It is definitely more therapeutic to focus on positive aspects of a situation and on the positive qualities of a person. A glass that is half-full is to be preferred over one that is half-empty. There is strong evidence to support the need to be optimistic and to speak in positive terms. A classic study showed that patients react much more favorably to being told that there is a 68% survival rate than that there is a 32% mortality rate.[22] Common sense tells us these statistics are the same. We can only speculate that in the first instance a patient focuses on the word "survival" and in the second only "mortality" is heard. The numbers are discounted.

It is important to keep in mind that in every case, our patients have definitively demonstrated their ability to survive, since if they had not, they would not be appearing in our offices at this time. One way or another, patients have surmounted the many challenges that are part of living in our rapidly changing society. We need to remember Theodore Rubin's insight that "The problem is not that there are problems. The problem is expecting otherwise and thinking that having problems is a problem."[23] It is how we react that matters. Once refocused on their healthy resources, patients will generally manage their problems and their lives in remarkably competent ways.

Making the Patient Responsible

Although the practitioner is available for help and support, responsibility for resolving all problems remains with the patient. The practitioner assumes the role of coach while the patient is the player who is held accountable for applying the strategies that have been discussed and for investigating various options. The practitioner expresses confidence in the patient's ability to gather and apply the resources necessary to arrive at a positive outcome. The patient is encouraged to stay in the "here and now," since fretting about the past or worrying about the future is not constructive. Things need to be taken one day at a time until there is some clear resolution. There is a mutual understanding that the situation will be discussed further at the next visit. The practitioner is interested in following all the developments. The time interval is clearly specified: "I want to see you next week and we will talk more." Although this approach works very well in many cases, patients do not always follow through as directed. Practitioners need not become frustrated. Instead we recommend applying the new scoring system and then redirecting the patient toward the desired goal.

Applying a New Scoring System

In evaluating patients' progress, we recommend applying an innovative scoring system for tracking new behavior. In the best behavioral tradition, it is designed to focus only on positive changes and ignore lapses and can be expected to produce excellent results. Since it has long been known that under stress people regress and are not able to apply most recently learned behavior,[24] lapses are to be ignored. Instead, patients are instructed to keep track of every time they engage in any new behavior. We are not interested in their recording failures (too many patients are stuck in their failure image), only instances of success. Patients are to give themselves credit (two points) every time they become aware of reacting, thinking, behaving, planning, or doing anything in a new way, that is, changing an old pattern.

Because it is hard to act in new ways or apply new behavioral techniques, doing it and recognizing doing it deserve two points. Patients must be informed that under stress it is normal and expected to react in old automatic ways. Certain behaviors have been over-learned and become a habit. Breaking habits is very difficult. The first and essential step to changing habitual behavior is to become aware that it is happening. Instructing patients not to get angry or abusive with themselves when they become aware that they have just reacted in an old way is the most important feature of the new scoring system. On the contrary, they get credit (one point) just for the recognition. One point is assigned for every time they notice that they have not taken advantage of an opportunity to react in a new way. Since this is scored as a success, it will provide reinforcement and motivation to apply the new behavior at the next opportunity. That is the reason for suggesting that patients give themselves credit (one point) every time they catch themselves doing something the old way.

Becoming conscious of behavior as it is occurring, starting to self-monitor, is a prerequisite for making lasting changes. By suggesting that the patient is doing something good (recognizing the behavior as it is happening), even when the patient is acting in the usual old way, we change the story. In this way we help patients to break the destructive cycle of feeling helpless and then abusing themselves for feeling that way. Instead, by changing the story before changing the target behavior, we put patients back in control, enhance their sense of self-efficacy, and induce positive change.

In the next chapter we will look at the content of the 15-minute therapy session and will introduce some further strategies and suggestions.

SUMMARY

Since illness or accidents exacerbate chronic conditions and sickness is often triggered by psychosocial stress, the practitioner should routinely ask all patients what is going on in their lives. The practitioner's interest indicates caring about the whole person. By making the inquiry routine, patients are educated to become aware of the interaction between their physical and psychological well-being.

If a patient is upset about the present situation the practitioner extends an invitation to talk. The practitioner tries to establish the significance of the event for the patient and accepts the patient's feelings. When a patient unexpectedly reacts emotionally during the course of an interview, the practitioner briefly explores the issue by BATHEing the patient. Patients' stories must be heard and reflected back with empathy, and then the limits must be challenged. By using the word "yet," the practitioner implies that the patient has the potential to change.

Small wins combat the patient's sense of being overwhelmed and allow patients to experience success. Incremental steps are effective in promoting change because they increase a patient's confidence. The practitioner engages the patient in a therapeutic contract by committing to follow the psychosocial context of the patient's life. Crises can generally be resolved within 6 or 8 weeks, which is also a good estimate for accomplishing grief work. The patient will do much of the work in writing and report the progress during regular visits.

Contracting to help the patient resolve the problem is one of the most affirming and therapeutic messages that can be conveyed. The patient now has a partner who has no agenda other than helping the patient through a difficult time. Accordingly, the patient feels less isolated and less overwhelmed by the problem. Often, when the patient's morale has been restored, the problems get resolved more expeditiously than expected. In difficult situations, the practitioner suggests that there might be options, invites the patient to consider consequences related to different choices, and suggests that applying "tincture of time," or deciding not to decide, is a viable option.

The patient learns that events have a symbolic significance (which is different for all people), that certain feelings are triggered by old memories, and that self-esteem, the sense of control, and the sense of being lovable are all affected by the interpretations of historical events. The practitioner points out that these old interpretations can affect current relationships. It is important not to generalize, but to take life one day at a time. Patients generally feel guilty about the past and anxious about the future, but dwelling on past hurts is not useful and assumptions about the future are usually wrong, so focusing in the present and engaging in active problem solving are therapeutic.

A three-step approach to problem solving involves asking what the patient is feeling, what the patient wants, and what the patient can do to maximize getting what he or she wants. The practitioner's support makes the patient feel more in control. The patient has a partner. The practitioner indicates confidence in the patient's ability to handle things. The patient feels less overwhelmed and resumes functioning in a healthier mode.

The practitioner focuses on the patient's strengths and acknowledges that the patient has survived similar situations, that support is available and can be asked for, and that the situation will be discussed further at the next visit. A scoring system that only records successes is instigated to reinforce new and more productive behavior.

References

1. McWhinney IR. Beyond diagnosis: an approach to the integration of behavioral science and clinical medicine. *N Eng J Med.* 1972; **287**: 384–7.
2. Bornstein PE, Clayton PJ. The anniversary reaction. *Dis Nerv Syst.* 1972; **33**: 470–2.
3. Cavenar JO, Nash JI, Maltbie AA. Anniversary reactions presenting as physical complaints. *J Clin Psychiatry.* 1978; **39**: 369–74.
4. Morgan CA, Hill S, Fox P, *et al.* Anniversary reactions in Gulf War veterans: a follow-up inquiry 6 years after the war. *Am J Psychiatry.* 1999; **156**(7): 1075–9.
5. McWhinney IR. *A Textbook of Family Medicine.* 2nd ed. New York: Oxford University Press; 1997. p. 31.
6. House JS, Landis KR, Umberson D. Social relationships and health. *Science.* 1988; **241**: 540–5.
7. Rogers CR. The necessary and sufficient conditions of therapeutic personality change. *J Consult Psychol.* 1957; **21**: 95–103.
8. Frank JD. Therapeutic components. In: Myers JM, (ed.) *Cures by Psychotherapy: What effects change?* New York: Praeger; 1984.
9. Stiles WB, Shapiro DA, Elliot, R. "Are all psychotherapies equivalent?" *Am Psychol.* 1986; **41**: 165–180.
10. Leichsenring F, Hiller W, Weissberg M, *et al.* Cognitive-behavioral therapy and psychodynamic psychotherapy: techniques, efficacy, and indications. *Am J Psychother.* 2006; **60**(3): 233–59.
11. Fishman DB. *The Case for Pragmatic Psychology.* New York: New York University Press; 1999. p. 5.
12. Frank JD. Psychotherapy: The restoration of morale. *Am J Psychiatry.* 1974; **131**: 271–4.

13. Peterson C, Seligman MEP, Vaillant GE. Pessimistic explanatory style as a risk factor for physical illness: a thirty-five-year longitudinal study. *J Per Soc Psychol.* 1988; **55**: 23–7.

14. Weick KE. Small wins: Redefining the scale of social problems. *Am Psychol.* 1984; **39**: 40–9.

15. Weick, op. cit. p. 45.

16. Caplan G. *Principles of Preventive Psychiatry.* New York: Basic Books; 1964.

17. Shem S. *The House of God.* New York: Dell Publishing; 1979.

18. Marsland AL, Prather AA, Petersen KL, *et al.* Antagonistic characteristics are positively associated with inflammatory markers independently of trait negative emotionality. *Brain Behav Immunol.* 2008; Jan 26. (Epub ahead of print).

19. Smith TW, MacKenzie J. Personality and risk of physical illness. *Ann Rev Clin Psychol.* 2006; **2**: 435–67.

20. Lawler-Row KA, Karremans JC, Scott C, *et al.* Forgiveness, physiological reactivity and health: the role of anger. *Int J Psychophysiol.* 2008; **68**(1): 51–8.

21. Freedman SR, Enright RD, Knutson JA. Progress report on the process model of forgiveness. In: Worthington EL Jr., (ed.) *Handbook of Forgiveness.* New York: Brunner- Routledge; 2005. pp. 393–406.

22. McNeil BJ, Pauker SG, Sox HC, *et al.* A. On the elicitation of preferences for alternative therapies. *N Eng J Med.* 1982; **306**: 1262.

23. Quoted by Brian Baker. "Quote of the day," (1 July 2001). Available from: www. quoteworld.org

24. Cohen S. Aftereffects of stress on human performance and social behavior: a review of research and theory. *Psychol Bull.* 1980; **88**: 82–108.

CHAPTER 6

Agenda for the Fifteen-Minute Counseling Session

The object of the interaction between the primary care practitioner and the patient in sessions devoted primarily to counseling is to promote change in the patient's behavioral, emotional, or cognitive reactions. In our view this can be defined as "psychotherapy," although we are acutely aware that both primary care practitioners and mental health professionals may be uncomfortable with this application of the term. The official dictionary definition of psychotherapy is simply treatment of mental or emotional or problems by psychological means.[1] In our view, when the therapeutic interaction with the practitioner has the intent of affecting the story patients tell themselves about the way things are and what is possible, that is psychotherapy.

In contrast, *counseling* suggests giving advice related to a particular situation. It fosters dependency and implies that the practitioner has more insight into a situation than the patient does. We would like to propose a compromise: that the practitioner be aware of making therapeutic interventions but refer to the process as counseling. Jay Fidler MD, a renowned psychiatrist and teacher, once remarked that the primary difference between just playing with a child and play therapy was what went on in the therapist's head.[2]

As long as the practitioner recognizes that the objective of the 15 minutes spent with the patient is therapeutic change, it can be presented to the patient as counseling, which may make both the patient and the practitioner more comfortable. The patient is scheduled for one or more brief counseling sessions to talk about an ongoing situation that is causing emotional discomfort. The practitioner's words and actions must be geared to promote the patient's sense of personal competence and connection to other people. The clinician intentionally supports strategies to help foster the patient's sense that the world is a reasonably reliable place and that even unfortunate circumstances can become learning experiences. This supports the patient's sense of coherence, the factor cited as most significant in promoting health.[3]

Basically, the practitioner uses a variety of techniques to help the patient adapt to the environment in ways that will improve mental and physical health. Let us look at how all this can be effectively incorporated into a 15-minute counseling session.

THE OPENING INQUIRY

It is important to start every session with an open question and let the patient talk about whatever the patient has been planning to say, has been thinking about, or finds most important to discuss at this time.

"What has been happening since I saw you?" "Tell me how you've been doing." "What sort of things have you been thinking about since last week?" "Tell me how you've been feeling and what's been going on." Any of these are good openers. Then it is important to let the patient talk without interrupting for about two or three minutes. This gives the patient the opportunity to reflect on what seems to be most important, currently. After about three minutes, it is critical to summarize what the patient has said in order to let him or her know that the practitioner has been really listening.

If the patient has not focused on events that have occurred since the previous visit, it is necessary to focus on the current situation and bypass elaborate background material. Asking "What is the most significant thing that's happened since I saw you last?" is a good way to redirect the conversation.

Next the practitioner may assess the patient's affect and inquire by reflecting, "You look less tense, how do you feel about what's been going on?" Or, "How have you been feeling since I saw you last?" In cases where patients are out of touch with their feelings or have a hard time expressing them, it is useful to summarize the feelings that appear to be underlying the story. "Sounds like you are disappointed (or discouraged, frustrated, annoyed), are you?" "I hear you blaming yourself, taking all the responsibility – do you feel guilty?"

After that, it is constructive to ask "What is the worst thing that has happened since last time?" It may be useful to explore what about the situation made it bothersome. It is the symbolic meaning of the event for the patient that is important. Finally, the practitioner asks how the patient feels about the way in which things were handled. An empathic response can be interjected whenever it seems appropriate.

It is also a good thing to focus on a success. More will be said about this in a later chapter. "Tell me about one thing that you handled well or that you feel good about." Or, "What's the best thing that has happened since I saw you?" The small wins, and the sense of mastery that grows with accomplishing them, are very important.

The sequence of these questions is deliberate. If it sounds familiar, it should. It is the BATHE sequence. It focuses the patient in the present and helps him or her to identify and express feelings. It looks at what was most troubling (cognitive assessment) and the way in which things were handled (behavioral assessment). It helps the patient develop an awareness that both good and bad things happen during each time period and that the patient makes choices in responding to them. These techniques are generic therapeutic interventions. We are promoting them because they are useful and easy to remember, and they work. They are certainly not the only way to do counseling, but they fit well into a brief-session framework and maximize the potential for positive outcome.

After going through the opening inquiry, it is important to make an empathic statement based on understanding the patient's experience during the intervening time since the last visit. If something positive has been reported, the practitioner might say, "I would think that you could feel very proud about having handled things in a new way." If the patient has not been successful, a useful intervention could be "It must be really discouraging and painful when you are trying so hard to cooperate, that things at home don't seem any different. Still, you get points for having made some changes. What do you think you might modify more?"

REPORTING ON HOMEWORK ASSIGNMENTS

After the opening inquiry, focus shifts to the homework assignment. "Did you create the list of options that might be available to you, and do you have it with you?" "Did you talk to your wife and let her know exactly what is troubling you?" "What did you learn from keeping the log of all the times that you got very upset?" "What sources of support were you able to come up with?" "Tell me about the list of the positive and negative potential outcomes related to going into your own business at this time." If the assignment has been done, the practitioner takes this as a positive sign that the patient is exhibiting responsible behavior and is taking control. The session can then center on what has been learned from the assignment or on one thing about which the patient is most concerned.

If the assignment has not been completed, the practitioner must accept the fact. It is imperative that practitioners not scold or try to induce guilt in the patient. Therapeutic interventions provide new responses to old patterns. The practitioner simply states that for some reason the patient chose not to do the assignment at this time, adding that it might be useful to identify the obstacles that were allowed to get in the way of doing the task and to recognize that there is always another opportunity:

"Mary, I can understand that you did not take the time to list the activities that really make you feel good. I wonder what makes it so hard for you to focus on things that you like. Do you want to do it for next week, or would you rather talk about it now?"

This approach communicates three important messages:
1. It is all right to be where you are. I accept you
2. You are making choices that have some meaning for you
3. However, there may be more constructive choices that you can make.

FACILITATING PATIENTS' ABILITY TO CHANGE

As we have said previously, people can and do make major changes in their behavior and in the way that they interpret the conditions of their lives (their story) but only when it is safe for them to do so and when they are ready. The brief counseling session can help to bring these positive conditions to pass.

Starting Where the Patient Is

The most important generic principle for making therapeutic interventions is that we have to start where the patient is (on his or her map). This is true in any type of teaching situation. In order to promote learning of any type, we first have to assess the level of the student's knowledge. If we were to present something that the student already knows, no learning would take place, since the student already has access to that information.[4] Conversely, if we start at a level more advanced than the student's background preparation, there would also be no learning because the new information would not be understood or incorporated. To be effective, we must start where any learner is at any given time. That means that we must accept our patients at their current levels of functioning, recognizing that as we do this without implied criticism, it facilitates patients' abilities to make small but positive changes.

Attentive Listening

Whenever the patient is speaking the practitioner's body language should communicate interest and attention. This can be done by maintaining eye contact while leaning toward the patient, refraining from writing, concentrating, nodding approvingly, and responding at appropriate times. It is valuable to notice the patient's affect as positive or negative material is being related. If there is a discrepancy between the affect (facial expression and body language) and the content of the patient's story, this can be gently pointed out: "I notice that you are smiling as you are telling me about all these terrible things that are happening." This is important feedback. Perhaps the patient is just nervous, or perhaps this incongruent affect is a long-term problem and one of the reasons that the patient has difficulty with personal relationships. Summarizing and reflecting back to the patient what has been heard demonstrates that the practitioner has been paying attention and has understood. Consequently, the patient is able to move on and to make changes.

Focusing the Patient in the Present

Since, by definition, we can only act at the current time, we recommend that patients generally be focused in the present. The only strong exceptions to this rule concern a history of sexual abuse or grief reactions where there is a need to review the past and sort out various feelings about the person, relationship, object, or position involved. We will say more about this later.

If a patient complains about how his mother treated him as a child, the practitioner can respond with some empathy but then wonder whether that is really relevant to how the patient presently treats his wife. What can the patient do to get more satisfaction from his current marriage? Also, what is it that the patient wants from his mother, now?

Probing for Feelings

Probably the most efficient therapeutic strategy is a two-step process of asking patients to identify feelings and then to accept these feelings as appropriate, given the underlying story.

When the patient relates what has been happening, good or bad, the practitioner inquires, "How did you feel about that?" It is interesting to observe reactions to this question. Patients often stop, look surprised at the direction of the conversation, and have to think for a moment before labeling the feeling. Many people are out of touch with their feelings, and most people are astonished when an authority figure expresses interest in their feelings. Often, patients do not respond with a label for a feeling but instead tell you what they thought or what someone else did. Let us look at an example:

> Mr. Graham is relating how he asked his wife to make some changes in her schedule to accommodate him and that she agreed without giving him any argument.
>
> Practitioner (breaking in): "How did you feel about that?"
>
> Patient: "I thought she would just refuse to go along with me."
>
> Practitioner: "I understand that, but how did it make you *feel*?"
>
> Patient: "I was surprised and pleased."
>
> Practitioner: "You really felt good."

In active listening it is useful to reflect understanding and acceptance by paraphrasing.

> A patient has just related that he tried hard to get his wife to listen to how he felt about having to go to her mother's for dinner every Saturday night. Instead of responding, she simply gave him "one of her looks" and left the room.
>
> Doctor: "So when Ethel walked away, how did you feel? Angry?" The patient nods.
>
> Doctor: "I can understand that. You must have felt awful."

Giving patients permission to feel the feelings that have been aroused requires a minimal investment of time, energy, and understanding. A patient is overheard saying to her friend in the waiting room, "My doctor told me that my feelings are legitimate, even if other people see things differently or feel some other way." Her affect would have been appropriate for announcing that she had just won the lottery.

Acceptance Must Precede Change

Once having elicited and accepted the patient's feelings, if the practitioner thinks it would be useful for the patient to become aware of how his or her behavior contributed to creating a bad situation, the next question might be "Tell me more about that. Then what did you decide to do?"

When asking for details or elaboration of events, we encourage focusing on the patient's behavior – what he or she thought and did and not stories about the thoughts and actions of other people. The underlying message is always that patients have choices. Indeed, they have power. Perhaps until now, the patient has not been aware of this.

Dealing with the Run-on Patient

Often patients find it difficult to stay within the structure prescribed by the practitioner. They will elaborate endlessly, or they will repeat themselves. When this occurs, it is essential that practitioners take a calming breath and then interrupt and summarize by saying, "Yes, you told me about _____. I know the details are important to you but tell me how it makes you *feel*." When patients talk about past events that cannot be changed, the practitioner might respond, "I hear how upset you are that things didn't work out. How does it make you feel *now*, and what might you do differently the next time?"

Getting patients to express guilt, anger, rage, or sadness helps them to accept their feelings and move on. Then they can examine options for dealing with matters now. They can change their stories of what is right and what is possible. They can make plans for how to handle things differently in the future.

Incorporating Medical Treatment

After the opening inquiry is completed, the practitioner may wish to follow up on any physical complaints. If there is an opportunity to "lay on hands," this is useful in helping the patient to connect physical and psychological symptoms. At this time, the practitioner may also discuss any changes in medications if they are part of the treatment. Medication is always an option to be used along with counseling, as previously discussed. The written prescription should not, however, be seen as part of the ritual offering that the practitioner presents to the patient, as discussed in Chapter 1. After the brief inquiry into the physical aspects, the practitioner focuses back on the psychosocial area: "All right, now let's talk about what you are going to do for next week."

COLLATERAL VISITS WITH FAMILY MEMBERS

As discussed in Chapter 1, one of the strong advantages the primary practitioner brings to the therapeutic encounter is the established relationship with the patient and the patient's family. A colleague, who is in solo private practice, reports the following case:

Gail, age 35, moved from Mississippi to New Jersey because of the demands of her husband's job. She is the daughter of alcoholic parents and has been suffering from an anxiety-depression syndrome for years. She has been treated with a variety of tranquilizers and antidepressants and is now struggling to adjust to life in a new community. Because of our inability to find a counselor with whom she felt comfortable, I, as her family practitioner, agreed to see her for some regular, brief sessions. Some of her problems focused on the unresponsiveness of her husband, Jim. She felt that he would not want to come in but agreed to ask him. I had seen him several times, in the office, with the children and for problems of his own, and was confident I had sufficient rapport to enable us to talk freely.

I began the interview by saying that I understood that it was his wife who had asked for help but that I felt it was important at this time to elicit his support. During the introductory comments, Jim assured me that he felt that he had a good relationship with his wife, even though they did not communicate much. It took very little to make him happy. Knowing that his wife and children were provided for and having some personal peace and quiet were all that he really needed. He realized that his wife needed more, such as a lovely home and an active social life. She also liked to be touched and caressed, but he was not "into" these things.

"How do you feel about these differences and the obvious lack of communication?" I asked.

He replied that he felt that they should improve their communication and, after some prompting, agreed that it was also probably important to their relationship to pay more attention to each other's interests but he "just hadn't thought much about it."

"For example," I asked, "what do you say when your wife says she wants to redecorate the dining room?"

"I tell her we don't have the money," he replied.

"Is that all?" I asked.

"Yes," he replied, "and the subject is dropped."

"Is there no way you could be more creative about this in order to satisfy your mutual interests?" I queried.

"Like what?" he wanted to know.

"For example, you might get a second job," I said.

"Or she might get a job," he replied quickly. This was something that Gail had wanted to do but was afraid her husband would not support. We agreed that this might solve several problems.

Moving on, I asked, "Do you remember your wife on Mother's Day?"

(I knew that he had this year.)

"Not usually," he said.

"How about birthdays?"

"Not usually. My family never made much of these things."

"How does she feel when you do remember her?" I asked.

"Oh, she loves it."

"Doesn't that give you pleasure also?" I wondered.

"Sure, but I just don't usually think about it."

"And in relation to sex, which you say you like, and touching, which you are not into, are you aware of some common differences between men and women in these areas?"

"Not really."

Here I mentioned some typical needs of women (often not understood by male partners) that were similar to those expressed by his wife. He seemed quite interested.

As we ended the interview (15 minutes exactly), he brightened up and said that this session had given him new ideas and much to think about and that he might be glad to talk with me again after he had time to do some homework.

In this case, the practitioner, by virtue of her established relationship with the family, in one visit was able to sensitize the husband to some very real problems experienced by his wife that under normal circumstances he would completely exclude from his map. The intervention proved to be extremely effective, and Gail's self-esteem increased dramatically as she experienced herself functioning well in her new job and having her husband act more attentive to her needs.

FORMATTING THE CHANGE PROCESS

Once patients recognize the need to change it is useful to focus on the patient's strengths, encourage new behavior, explore options, and employ some simple formulas to guide the process.

Focus on the Patient's Strengths

The essence of supportive therapeutic interventions is to restore patients' faith in their own capacity to take charge of their lives in a productive and satisfying way. Every difficult situation is a variation on some previous situation. If patients had not survived these earlier traumas, they would not be presenting themselves at this time. It is the practitioner's job to remind patients about having overcome past obstacles. This enhances the sense of coherence.[3] If patterns have consistently been destructive, then patients must be encouraged to make small changes in the ways that they would normally react in order to achieve more positive outcomes.

Each of us has a rather limited behavioral repertoire. In any situation, there is some way that we naturally respond because that is what we have previously learned to do. We tell ourselves the story that this will work. When we do not get the expected or desired result, we often redouble our efforts and keep doing whatever we are doing, longer and harder, becoming more and more frustrated when we continue to fail to achieve our ends. We have what psychologists call a limited *response set*. It is not necessary to explore why and how these behavioral patterns developed, but to focus on what the patient gains from maintaining the dysfunctional behavior. If this turns out to be nothing or pain, then we can encourage patients to change their behavior. We specifically encourage acting in some new and different ways, to develop a broader response set, and to monitor the result.

Exploration of Options

In many cases people who are caught in a painful emotional situation are not aware that there are always options. Naturally, each potential choice has consequences, but awareness of the power to choose (even if only our attitude) makes us feel less impotent and overwhelmed.

In the early 1960s, Stanley Milgram[5] experimentally studied obedience to authority. In a disguised learning task, an experimenter demanded that subjects apply shock to a stooge, who pretended to be adversely affected by this treatment. Subjects routinely followed orders although they showed discomfort, especially after passing into a range of shock marked "danger." A movie was made in which the interactions among subject, experimenter, and stooge could be observed. Although most subjects performed as directed when they were simply told, "You must continue with the experiment," in those cases where the experimenter added, "You have no choice," subjects invariably stopped, thought for a few moments, and then said something to the effect that of course they had a choice. They could walk out. And then they walked out. It seemed that just having the word "choice" mentioned made them aware that there were options.

Most people looking back on what seem to have been serious mistakes made during turning points in their lives will say that it never occurred to them that there were other options. There are always options if we take the time to look for them. It is helpful to remind patients that they do have choices, one of which is not to decide at that particular time; to choose not to choose, at least for the present. The practitioner suggests that the patient lists a variety of options as a homework assignment and comes back to discuss things further.

Behavioral Options

In Chapter 5 we introduced the following sequence:
1. What are you feeling?
2. What do you want?
3. What can *you* do about it?

This sequence helps to shift the responsibility for taking effective action to the patient. Rather than fretting about someone else's behavior over which they have no control, patients focus on novel approaches for getting their own needs met. Inviting patients to respond to situations in a different way promotes new behavior. If a wife cannot stop her husband from excess drinking, she can decide that since there is nothing that she can do to affect his behavior, she can change hers. She will stop arguing and fighting with him, stop aggravating herself about it, and engage instead in some activity that she enjoys. She may even decide to go to Al-Anon and get some support for herself. In this case, the patient chooses an alternate way of responding to a situation. The situation remains the same, but her perception of it and her response to it have changed. As a result, she feels less overwhelmed. Moreover, since she has disturbed the homeostasis of the conflict in their relationship, the husband's behavior may ultimately also change.

Four Options in a Bad Situation

Patients are taught that there are four healthy options for handling a bad situation:
1. leaving it
2. changing it
3. accepting it as it is (and getting support elsewhere)
4. reframing it (interpreting the situation differently).

Option 1

When considering leaving a situation, be it a relationship, job, or any intolerable circumstance, patients should be encouraged to assess the best and worst possible outcomes should they leave. They can then be instructed to weigh the likelihood of each of these occurrences. Having a specific strategy to employ will give these patients a sense of competence and power in making the decision. If they decide to leave, they can be encouraged to plan the timing, obtain needed resources and other support, and practice what they want to say when informing the various affected parties. It is important that they consider contingency plans and explore all the relevant details. For instance, a patient with a chronic medical condition should think carefully about leaving a job and losing health insurance coverage without being certain that a new position will provide adequate benefits. Behavioral rehearsal of this kind fosters a high order of adaptive coping. These behavioral preparations, or potential scripts, constitute useful homework assignments, to be brought back to the practitioner for discussion.

Option 2

In considering whether a situation can be changed, patients need to look at what resources are available and what strategies might be employed. Has the patient communicated clearly with the powers-that-be regarding the level of dissatisfaction? Can the patient clearly define the problem and make suggestions for a positive resolution? Behavioral change on the part of the patient may ultimately change the responses of significant other people, thereby changing the situation. Sometimes outside pressure can be brought to bear on the situation, and often time alone will effect a change. In this case, it may be appropriate to accept the situation as it is for the moment.

Option 3

Accepting a situation as it is and not aggravating oneself by thinking that it should be different constitute a very constructive option. People make themselves miserable when they continually tell themselves the story that the circumstances they find are not as they should be. It is necessary to accept the fact that at any given time, things are the way they are. Given acceptance of that fact if, for instance, one's job is tedious, outside activities that are interesting and satisfying can be encouraged. Support groups, close friends, and exercise programs are all means of relieving stress. Taking pride in the quality of one's work and interactions with other people can also help to make accepting the situation more pleasant. Recognizing that time will probably bring change, it is constructive to make oneself comfortable while waiting for something to occur. It always does, usually in unexpected ways.

Option 4

Changing the interpretation of a situation (i.e., reframing it or looking at it in a new way) is the most creative and satisfying way of dealing with difficult circumstances. When patients use novel ways of reinterpreting situations, when they change the story about the meaning of the circumstances, they are adapting in a growth-producing fashion and enhancing their mental and physical health.[6] Every difficult task can be viewed as an opportunity to gain skill and experience, to learn something of value, or to become stronger or more flexible. Seen in this light, the situation can prove more valuable and rewarding than had things worked out as originally desired or planned. It is the meaning that we attribute to a situation that determines how we feel about it, as shown by the following example:

> Barbara D. was a patient with multiple problems, including severe back pain, generally unresponsive to treatment. She was moderately depressed and very concerned about her demanding husband and also about her mother-in-law, in whose home they lived. When Barbara complained that her husband "should not

be so demanding," the practitioner suggested that this could be reframed to provide Barbara the opportunity to practice her assertiveness skills. The change in Barbara's attitude proved remarkable. She simply glowed the following week while reporting how she had handled several situations that previously would have left her feeling impotent rage. Not only that, but her back pain had almost entirely resolved.

The Problem Always Belongs to the Patient

Perhaps the most important factor to keep in mind when doing counseling in the 15-minute framework is that the problem belongs to the patient. The process of medical education predisposes the practitioner to take on and solve problems. The first step in problem solving is to accurately define the problem. In this case the problem must be defined as the patient's reaction. The practitioner cannot afford to get intimately involved in the details of the situation or understand the exact etiology or even the specific effect of the circumstances on all the people involved. The practitioner is not responsible for solving the patient's problem. Rather, the practitioner's responsibility is limited to supporting the patient so that the patient can identify the specific problem that may be underlying the experienced stress, making the patient aware that this problem is contributing to the feelings of illness that he or she is experiencing, and encouraging the patient to explore potential solutions for the problem, as in the following example:

Mrs. K., a 30-year-old Asian mother of a three-month-old boy, is in the office for the third time in two weeks. She is complaining about feeling tired all the time, with headaches and some dizziness. She says that her body feels strange. On previous visits it has been determined that she is not anemic. Mrs. K. is delighted with her baby and reports that her husband is very supportive and concerned, and that her mother is living with them and helping to care for the child. As he leaves the room after an uneventful exam, the practitioner wonders what is really going on. He speculates whether having her mom there is making the patient feel competitive for the baby's attention. Perhaps the lifestyle change triggered by the birth is causing a conflict. Armed with specific theories, the doctor reenters the exam room. "Mrs. K., I really am sorry that you feel so bad. I found nothing during my exam to cause me any concern. Still, something is causing your symptoms. What do you think it might be?"

At first, the patient looks at him blankly and says nothing. The practitioner inquires, "What is going on in your life?" Hesitantly, the patient discloses that her mother is planning to return to Hong Kong and leave her to manage the baby alone. The practitioner asks how she feels about that. She admits that she is afraid to function independently and does not want to be cut off from her mom and the outside world and feels inadequate to care for her son. The doctor explains how anxiety can produce physical symptoms. He then focuses on supporting the patient, accepting her feelings and asking her to think about what skills she must learn while her mother is still there. Another appointment is made. His plan is to enhance her sense of self-efficacy (*see* Chapter 3) in an effort to convince her that she is capable of performing as a mother. He will motivate her by focusing on how important this is to her and how she can gain the necessary skill and confidence. He will also continue to be there for her and provide support and advice.

When the practitioner communicates the expectation that the patient, having identified the problem, will find some constructive resolution, a positive message is conveyed. The patient is empowered. The practitioner agrees to be part of the process, support initiatives, and make suggestions for strategies that can be employed, but it is clear to both parties that the patient has the responsibility to deal with the problem (which, by definition, is expected to yield to resolution).

THE PRACTITIONER'S ACCEPTANCE IS PART OF THE TREATMENT

In discussing stressful elements of the patient's life, the practitioner's attention and calm acceptance of the circumstances have a beneficial effect on the patient.

Accepting the Patient

The patient feels accepted as a person. The practitioner's interest is seen as supportive. Reflections by the practitioner help to make the patient feel competent. The patient feels valued, understood, and connected. The absence of criticism helps to counteract discouragement and self-doubt.

Accepting the Situation

By calmly accepting the situation, the practitioner becomes a role model for the patient. Together they look at a set of circumstances that, however unfortunate and difficult, first needs to be accepted and then needs to be handled. Just labeling the situation as a problem will change it. Problems lend themselves to a variety of solutions, some of which are better than others. There is now a direction for thinking constructively.

Accepting the Patient's Reaction

The practitioner's acceptance of the patient's reaction to the situation is therapeutic. Stating "This must be very difficult for you!" communicates to the patient that anyone would be stressed in similar circumstances. Usually it focuses the patient back on his or her strength: "Actually, I'm doing O.K., all things considered."

Changing the Underlying Story

In previous chapters we introduced the idea that patients' assumptive world view is the story that they tell themselves about how the world operates. None of us experiences the world directly. Rather, we experience subjective representations of circumstances that we filter through our visual, auditory, tactile, or other senses and then interpret, based on our previous experience. We delete cues that do not fit into our previous frame of reference as though there was no such territory on our map. The resulting model of the world, the story that we create, determines what choices and limitations we think we have or that we impose on ourselves. When we mistake our limited representation of the world for the real world, we limit our options.

When the practitioner assumes that there are more options than patients are seeing (and it is not necessary for the practitioner to be able to generate them), patients begin to expand their models of the world, and their stories may allow for new interpretations. Patients start to include a variety of options and reexamine their limitations. The whole idea of the therapeutic intervention is to open patients up to existing possibilities and to invite them to look at their world, including themselves, in new ways. Patients become aware that they have choices.

Enhancing the Patient's Self-esteem

Being open to possibilities is probably the hallmark of mental health. An impressive amount of data shows that positive illusions, rather than accurate contact with reality, lead to a sense of well-being and mental health characterized by the ability to care for others and do creative work.[7,8] As discussed previously, having a positive view of the self, an exaggerated belief in the ability to control the environment, and an optimistic view of the future is protective for mental and physical health. The practitioner's job is to help patients focus on positive aspects of themselves and their lives. When the patient expresses doubt about the ability to overcome some obstacle, the practitioner's confidence can be expressed by saying something like "You may have had problems with this in the past, but *I* see no reason that you cannot accomplish this now."

THE ROLE OF ADVICE

Practitioners are notorious for giving advice, and patients generally ask to be advised. They feel dependent, look up to the practitioner, and often want to be told what to do because they are afraid to make decisions or rely on their own abilities. Since they feel inadequate, they also feel out of control of their own destinies. Giving specific advice is always less effective than focusing patients back on their own resources, with appropriate instructions for developing alternatives. When the practitioner gives advice, the implication is that he or she has a better understanding of the patient's problems and options than the patient has. This does not empower patients. On the other hand, making patients aware of their own abilities and encouraging them to exercise their options is both therapeutic and practical. There are, however, certain suggestions that the practitioner can make. These focus primarily on the process of dealing with problems.

Behavioral Management of Children

Raising responsible children and enjoying the process requires that parents develop specific skills. Practitioners can be very helpful in response to particular behavioral problems that parents relate. However, even in the absence of specific complaints as part of well-child or routine visits, we encourage practitioners to promote the following principles: rewarding children's good behavior and ignoring bad behavior, setting strict limits on unacceptable behavior without making threats, using time-out to achieve control when children are uncooperative, allowing children to express feelings of all kinds but not allowing destructive behavior, and creating opportunities for children to make choices whenever possible.

Rewarding Good Behavior

When patients complain about their children's behavior, they can be advised to apply behavioral principles. Primarily, this means reinforcing (rewarding) good behavior and extinguishing (ignoring) inappropriate behavior. Parents are encouraged to try to "catch" their children "doing something right"[9] and then to reward them. Patients must understand that attention is a reward, so acknowledging good behavior consistently instead of focusing attention on bad behavior promotes rapid improvement.

Setting Limits

Parents must set strict limits on completely unacceptable or dangerous behavior. They should be instructed to be firm without making threats so that their children understand that the parents really mean what they say. When a parent says, "If you do such and such, I will punish you," it implies that the child has an option. The child has to decide whether doing the forbidden thing is worth the spanking, provided that Mother will actually follow through with the threat, which perhaps she will not. If, on the other hand, a clear statement is made, "I don't want you to do that," or "Stop that now!" there is no argument. In general, young children try to please their parents. Limits must be set reasonably and enforced consistently. If necessary, parents can be instructed to remove a child from a situation physically, firmly but gently, and to instigate *time-out*, a respite in a boring place, as an effective form of discipline.

Using Time-out

Any time a child is out of control, not behaving according to set standards, or failing to respect another person's rights, time-out becomes a way to allow him or her to contain emotions without damaging the self or others. The child is escorted to a predetermined area (someplace considered "boring" – not the child's bedroom) that has a door that can be closed. The child is told that once he or she is quiet, back in control, and willing to cooperate, time-out will be suspended. Depending on the age of the child, two to 15 minutes is usually sufficient to have the child calm down. Time-out is very effective if applied consistently.

Expressing Feelings

It is essential that parents encourage children to express feelings rather than engage in destructive behavior, such as physical violence. Negative feelings must be allowed as well as positive ones. Children need to learn that becoming frustrated, angry, sad, confused, or cranky is part of the normal human experience. When children make statements such as "I hate you," this needs to be interpreted as "Right this instance, you are very angry with me." This can be followed with "I'm sorry that you feel this way, but in spite of the fact that you think it would be fun, I cannot allow you to . . ." Children must learn that conflict is part of life but cannot be allowed to become physical.

Giving Children Choices

Parents are encouraged to give children choices whenever possible. The opportunity to practice making decisions that impact one's life, from an early age, helps establish a positive sense of self-esteem and self-efficacy. For example, after a long day of shopping, one of our patients had a hard time getting a tired and cranky three-year-old to wash his hands before dinner until she asked him whether he would rather wash his hands in the sink or in the bath tub. He laughed, chose the tub, and immediately complied.

Dealing with Teenagers

Adolescents must be allowed to take part in making decisions that affect their lives and must also be held responsible for living up to their commitments. Parents are encouraged to discuss reasonable limits with their teenage children and to negotiate joint agreements on acceptable rules. When a teenager does not follow through on a commitment, this must be addressed as a problem and renegotiated. In this way, the young person's self-esteem and self-control are fostered while the parent can relinquish the role of police officer.

Parents are cautioned not to get into power struggles with their adolescent children. In a power struggle both parent and child lose, since when the parent wins the battle, the child's sense of control and self-esteem are compromised, generally leading to more destructive behavior. It is more constructive to jointly discuss options and to give the teenager an opportunity to decide between several acceptable alternatives. When parents treat teenagers as responsible individuals, express trust in their judgment, and respect their privacy, this information becomes part of the adolescents' sense of self, and they can be expected to act accordingly. It is foolish to minimize the dangers of peer pressure on teenagers to experiment with drugs and sex and to engage in other risky behavior. However, parents have the power to make their children feel wanted, valued, and respected. This will result in adolescents developing the self-esteem and social skills to generally deter them from engaging in self-destructive behavior.

Recommending Resources

Many useful books are available to help parents learn the above techniques. The classics, *Parent Effectiveness Training* by T. Gordon[10] and *How to Talk So Kids Will Listen & How to Listen So Kids Will Talk*[11] and *How to Talk So Teens Will Listen. How to Listen So Teens will Talk*[12] by Faber and Mazlish are practical and effective. *The New Peoplemaking*, by Virginia Satir,[13] is a very readable and useful guide for managing children. All these are available in paperback. Parents can be encouraged to go to their libraries and browse or to look for paperbacks available in their local stores. The psychology/self-help sections of most bookstores have an incredible array of helpful inexpensive manuals directed at specific problems. Relevant books can be read and discussed in subsequent sessions. The practitioner can save much time when patients get information from books and then come back to discuss their reactions. This is called *bibliotherapy*.[14] Appendix B lists helpful books that can be recommended to patients for this purpose.

Regardless of the recommendations made, it is important that the practitioner not forget to give the usual empathic support. "It must be very difficult to manage a teenager (three-year-old, two active children, or whatever) when you have all these other things going on in your life. Let's talk more about that next time."

Assertiveness Training

Patients should be encouraged to become appropriately assertive. In dealing with other people, patients must learn to see themselves and their desires as neither more nor less important than the desires of other people. Practitioners should advise patients to send "I" messages, learn to state their feelings, ask for what they want, and give their reactions to other people's behavior. For example: "When you ignore me when I walk into the room, I feel discounted" or "When I make dinner, and you don't come when I call you, I feel very angry." Saying "I don't like it when you don't do what you say you are going to do" is much more effective in getting another person to follow through on a promise than saying "You *never* do *anything* you say you are going to do!"

Patients are encouraged to persevere and insist that their rights be respected. Again, there are several books that the practitioner can recommend: *Your Perfect Right* by Alberti and Emmons[15] and *When I Say No, I Feel Guilty* by Manuel Smith[16] are outstanding examples. As before, the encouragement and interest coming from the practitioner are more important than reading self-help books. However, the support of the practitioner in conjunction with the outside reading is the most effective strategy.

Taking Care of Oneself

One prescription that we encourage the practitioner to give patients is the instruction to be kind to, to be gentle with, and to take good care of themselves. When patients are experiencing periods of high stress, they must be told to modify the demands they make on themselves. They cannot expect to function at optimal levels and will feel much better if they lower their expectations. Moreover, they can give themselves credit for dealing with a difficult situation.

Patients should be advised to give themselves treats, to take breaks, and to plan desirable activities on a regular basis so that they always have something to look forward to. It is important that they work on maintaining supportive relationships with people they enjoy and make the time to visit or at least keep in touch by phone. The message here is "You are important, and your happiness and sense of well-being are also important and must be a priority for you."

Patients are encouraged to learn stress management techniques, such as controlled breathing, progressive relaxation, and meditation. They need to be encouraged to exercise regularly, choosing a modality they enjoy, and also need to learn to monitor and change their thinking patterns.

Distinguishing Among Thoughts, Feelings, and Behavior

It is important to teach patients to distinguish among thoughts, feelings, and behavior. Thoughts are constant internal messages that are often not noticed but are powerful enough to create our most intense emotions. Thoughts are the stories we use to describe the world to ourselves and to compare our perception of the way things are with the way we would like them to be. Based on these judgments, we then decide if things are good or bad, painful, dangerous, or just not as they should be.[17,18] In this way, our thoughts determine the way that we feel about a situation, another person, or ourselves.

Feelings constitute an automatic emotional response based on our judgments and interpretations. Feelings must be accepted, because they cannot be controlled directly. Given our interpretation of a situation (based on our story) we feel as we do. Cognitive therapy consists of challenging the underlying value judgments and assumptions that determine what we think. When we learn to modify our thought processes (i.e., edit our stories), moderate our expectations, and change our judgments, our feelings change.

Behavior is voluntary. We choose how we will act. When we are in touch with our feelings, we can learn to control our behavior. Our behavior is probably the only thing in life we can control. Our behavior should aim to get us what we want and enable us to present ourselves to the world as we wish to be seen. A practitioner can be very angry with a patient but keep the feeling hidden by choosing his or her words carefully in order not to intimidate the patient and to maximize the patient's cooperation.

In a brief counseling session the practitioner can help the patient to make distinctions between thoughts, feelings, and behavior; challenge irrational thoughts (the absolutes, unrealistic expectations, generalizations, and unfounded prognostications); accept feelings; and focus on behavior that can be changed.

Taking Responsibility for Our Feelings

The last piece of specific advice we suggest that practitioners offer patients is that it is useful to take responsibility for our own feelings. Few people realize that no one can actually make us feel anything. We feel the way we do as an automatic response to our interpretation of a given situation. A change in the interpretation changes the feeling. For example, if we presume that *all* practitioners reading this book will agree with our approach to therapy, we will feel very badly if some reviewers object to parts of the text or express reservations. On the other hand, if we hope simply that a few clinicians will find this book helpful and successfully use the techniques that we are proposing, we will be delighted when some people let us know that they are finding it useful.

Our current level of self-esteem, expectations for the future, and general outlook determine how we feel and not what actually happens to us. It is the practitioner's task to make the patient aware that we make ourselves feel hurt, angry, frustrated, and rejected by the stories we tell ourselves about what has happened or is going to happen. The resulting feelings we generate are often painful. If we are going to turn off the pain, we must first become aware of what we are feeling, decide what about the situation is so troubling, and then modify those feelings by reinterpreting (revising the story of) our circumstances.

Homework

The specific homework task for the intervening time between sessions is jointly determined. The patient makes a contract with the practitioner agreeing to keep a journal, prioritize problems, find a specific book, engage in regular exercise, and in general initiate and monitor changes in behavior and the resultant consequences.

It is important that the time spent with the practitioner be devoted to building skills that the patient can use to change interactions with the significant others in his or her life. It is up to the patient to chart his or her own progress during the intervening time. Homework assignments, particularly writing tasks, have been shown to be highly effective in promoting therapeutic change.[19–21] The outcome of the homework will be discussed at the next session. Knowing that the practitioner will be expecting a report helps motivate the patient to follow through on the assignment, as shown by the following example:

> Carol G. is a 22-year-old white female and mother of two children (three and five years old) who is currently living with a boyfriend; she came to the office complaining of two weeks of dizziness. She seemed totally overwhelmed by the multiple problems in her life. For a homework assignment the practitioner suggested that Carol keep a

journal and record all instances of dizziness and the particular circumstances when they occurred. Returning the following week, Carol was able to recognize that her dizziness occurred primarily when she felt most out of control, dealing with her estranged husband, her in-laws, her child's teacher, and her mother.

For the following week she was given the assignment to "do one thing nice for yourself." The resulting change was dramatic. Carol had decided to have lunch with a friend, leaving her mother to baby sit. She and her friend talked through her problems and after sleeping soundly that night, Carol contacted a lawyer to start divorce proceedings.

ENDING THE SESSION

Ending the session on time is important for both practitioner and patient. It is an affirmation of the patient's ability to cope and to apply the strategies discussed in the session. It also ensures that the contract is valid and that the practitioner intends to follow through, thereby securing the sense of connection. It is beneficial to hold encounters with the patient to a quarter of an hour. In general, during a regular medical appointment or brief counseling session the limited time spent focusing on the psychological aspects of the patient's situation allows only one or two major points to be made. Our experience has been that this has a powerful positive effect. Since persons under stress have a limited capacity to concentrate and process new information, dealing with only one or two issues prevents information overload. It also tends to make the problem seem less overwhelming.

At the end of the allotted time, the practitioner should make an honest comment acknowledging a positive aspect of how the patient is dealing with the situation and to "wish that there was more time." (This lets the patient know that the practitioner values the contact.) Stating that he or she is looking forward to continuing the discussion at the next scheduled session assures the connection. The patient is instructed to call if something serious occurs in the meantime.

In general, the patient should be allowed to talk for 12 minutes out of the 15. Brief comments from the practitioner should keep the patient focused on one or two tasks that can be used as preparation for the next session. Dealing with only one or two issues during a particular session prevents the patient from becoming confused or overloaded. Thus the practitioner is teaching a process while treating a person.

Results Over Time

Now let us look at a case that was handled by a young practitioner under our supervision and is typical of the effective outcome that can be expected over time:

Daniel G., a 16-year-old white male, presented at the Family Practice Center, on a Tuesday afternoon in late November, complaining of dizzy spells. The previous Sunday he had felt light-headed and dizzy and actually passed out. The patient said there had been two or three previous episodes but denied recent fever, palpitations, or chest pain.

Daniel and his mother had recently moved into the area to live with his grandmother. He related that he had no friends and was mostly interested in his baseball card collection. He admitted that he felt badly about the fact that he had no father and that his mother was crippled and confined to a wheelchair. The patient revealed that he wanted to become a carpenter.

A physical examination, including a complete neurological exam, was normal, allowing the practitioner, for the moment, to rule out an impending catastrophic medical event. His impression was vasovagal syncopal episodes. For completeness, routine laboratory tests were ordered, but the practitioner was more concerned that this patient needed emotional support. Daniel G. was a shy, sensitive individual with many emotional problems and no one to talk to. This made him feel very depressed. The practitioner made a contract for follow-up in one week with the expressed intention of seeing the patient for counseling.

In the course of having blood drawn, the patient became dizzy and his blood pressure dropped to 60/40, reinforcing the contention that this patient's symptoms were manifestations of vagal activity. In a half-hour his blood pressure had returned to normal, and the patient was released.

Daniel returned the following week. There had been no further episodes of dizziness. He then started to talk about his home situation. There was a horrendous history of abuse on the part of a man living with the mother and constant moves. The practitioner gave support and focused the patient on the present situation. Daniel had made a new friend in school and felt good about that, but he expressed a desire to transfer to vocational school. The practitioner said he would look into the possibility.

A contract was made to see the patient regularly once each week for 15-minute sessions. During the third session, Daniel appeared nervous and depressed. His affect was rather flat. He seemed to have nothing much to say. He wondered why the practitioner was interested in seeing him. The practitioner said that he enjoyed talking with Daniel and would like to help him to learn to make other friends and focus on planning his life.

By the fourth week, the patient was much more cooperative. He was happy about a project in school and spontaneously started to share some of his interests. During Christmas week, the patient canceled his appointment. He arrived early in January complaining of a head cold but feeling much happier. It was during this session that the patient revealed a history of sexual abuse occurring several years previously and expressed how happy he was to be receiving counseling. The practitioner assured Daniel that it was not his fault that he had been abused and acknowledged that it must have been awful for him. This seemed to relieve the boy. The subject was brought up several weeks later but seemed to have lost its impact.

Over the next several months, Daniel was seen regularly for counseling every other week. In time, he became involved with the golf club at school and made one close friend. He was treated for a sore throat and some nose bleeds and developed a very relaxed and trusting relationship with his doctor. After about one year, his afternoon job prevented him from attending his sessions regularly. A sports physical clearing him for team participation is the last item in the chart. When Daniel moved away at 17½ years of age, he appeared to be a rather confident, reasonably well-adjusted young man who was clear about his goals and directed toward achieving them.

SUMMARY

When starting a counseling session, the opening inquiry should focus on the present situation, a report on the homework assignment, and the best and worst things that transpired in the interim since the previous visit. The practitioner always starts where the patient is and communicates interest through attentive listening. Questions should generally probe for feelings and what the patient personally did in response to circumstances. Medication, laying-on of hands through examinations, and collateral visits with family members constitute other options that can be exercised.

In general, patients should be focused in the present. They are encouraged to focus on what they are feeling, what they want, and what they can do about it. Four healthy options for handling a painful situation are leaving it, changing it, accepting it with additional support, and reframing or reinterpreting (changing the story) it in a positive manner. Practitioners must gently set limits on the amount of detail or repetition that a patient presents. The practitioner is supportive of the patient. The practitioner's acceptance is therapeutic; however, the problem continues to belong to the patient. The practitioner accepts the patient, the situation, and the patient's reaction to the situation but assumes that there are always options that have yet to be considered.

In giving advice, the practitioner focuses on the process of dealing with problems, rather than their content. Advice may be given regarding behavioral strategies for managing children, becoming assertive, and taking care of the self. The practitioner points out the differences among thoughts, feelings, and behavior and how thoughts (judgments and/or stories) may be modified, with resulting emotional changes. Patients are held responsible for their own feelings. At the end of the session the practitioner extends the contract through the assignment of homework and the expectation that the patient will return to report on the accomplishment of a particular task. During the 15 minute session the patient should speak for about 12 minutes, with brief comments from the practitioner focusing on constructive elements. Time limits should be strictly adhered to. A successful counseling relationship with a teenager spanning over a year's time is described.

References

1. American Psychological Association. *Psychotherapy.* (n.d.). WordNet® 3.0. Available from: http://dictionary.reference.com/browse/psychotherapy (accessed 29 February 2008).
2. Fidler J. Lecture. Rutgers Community Mental Health Center Group Psychotherapy Training Program, 1974.
3. Antonovsky A. *Health, Stress, and Coping.* San Francisco: Jossey-Bass; 1979.
4. Whitman NA, Schwenk TL. *Preceptors as Teachers: a guide to clinical teaching.* Salt Lake City, Utah: University of Utah School of Medicine Press; 1984.
5. Milgram S. Behavioral study of obedience. *J Abnorm Soc Psychol.* 1963; **67**: 371–8.
6. Vaillant GE. Natural history of male psychologic health: effects of mental health on physical health. *N Eng J Med.* 1979; **301**: 1249–54.
7. Taylor SE, Kemeny ME, Reed GM, *et al.* Psychological resources, positive illusions, and health. *Am Psychol.* 2000; **55**(1): 99–109.
8. Gana K, Alaphilippe D, Bailly N. Positive illusions and mental and physical health in later life. *Aging Ment Health.* 2004; **8**(1): 58–64.
9. Blanchard K, Johnson S. *The One Minute Manager.* New York: William Morrow & Co.; 1982.
10. Gordon T. *Parent Effectiveness Training: the proven program for raising responsible children.* New York: Crown Publishing Group; 2000.
11. Faber A, Mazlish E. *How to Talk So Kids Will Listen: how to listen so kids will talk.* New York: William Morrow and Co.; 1999.
12. Faber A, Mazlish E. *How to Talk so Teens Will Listen: how to listen so teens will talk.* New York: HarperCollins; 2005.
13. Satir V. *The New Peoplemaking.* Palo Alto, CA: Science and Behavior Books; 1988.
14. Jamison C, Scogin F. The outcome of cognitive bibliotherapy with depressed adults. *J Consult Clin Psychol.* 1995; **63**(4): 644–50.
15. Alberti RE, Emmons M. *Your Perfect Right.* 8th ed. San Luis Obispo, CA: Impact Publishers; 2001.
16. Smith MJ. *When I Say No, I Feel Guilty.* New York: Bantam Press; 1985.
17. Beck AT. *Cognitive Therapy and Emotional Disorders.* New York: New American Library; 1979.
18. Ellis A. *Overcoming Destructive Beliefs, Feelings, and Behaviors: new directions for rational emotive behavior therapy.* Amherst, NY: Prometheus Books; 2001.
19. Cameron LD, Nicholls G. Expression of stressful experiences through writing: effects of a self-regulation manipulation for pessimists and optimists. *Health Psychol.* 1998; **17**(1): 84–92.
20. Smyth JM, Stone AA, Hurewitz A, *et al.* Effects of writing about stressful experiences on symptom reduction in patients with asthma or rheumatoid arthritis: a randomized trial. *JAMA.* 1999; **281**(14): 1304–9.
21. Burns DD. Homework facilitates positive changes in depression. *J Consult Clin Psychol.* 2000; **68**: 46–56.

CHAPTER 7

Therapeutic Interventions for Difficult Patient Situations

Now it is time to focus on some of the more difficult patient encounters. There are patients who are hard to treat because they are hard to be with. There are hostile patients, addicted patients, anxious and depressed patients who may or may not take medication, chronic pain patients, and suicidal patients, to mention only a few. How can we relate to them? And what do we do with those patients suffering from the current "disease of the month," whether chronic fatigue, fibromyalgia, or another somatization disorder? Can we really do anything for them? What is more important, can we help them without feeling put upon – without feeling totally depleted and less able to relate with genuine empathy to other patients?

Also, what, if anything, can we do to treat children and adolescents reacting to challenging circumstances of their lives? First, how do we get them to talk? Then, what do we do with the information?

A word of caution is in order. The techniques outlined in this chapter build on previous material. The practitioner must acquire a thorough understanding and a reasonable level of comfort using our supportive techniques in routine patient care before applying these specific approaches to the care of their most difficult patients. Providing supportive psychotherapy is a skill that needs to be practiced consistently and applied broadly to all patients.

REACTING TO DIFFICULT PATIENTS

Over 30 years ago Groves[1] wrote an article provocatively entitled "Taking Care of the Hateful Patient," in which he developed four stereotypes of particularly difficult patient personalities and behavioral categories. The four stereotypes are dependent clingers, manipulative help-rejecters, entitled demanders, and self-destructive deniers. Such individuals precipitate negative feelings on the part of practitioners, who feel depleted by the need to provide endless emotional supplies without achieving any objective positive outcome. After grouping differences and similarities, Groves developed specific approaches for dealing with each of these patient types.

Our approach is much simpler. We start with the notion that each patient is behaving in the best possible way, for this patient, at this time and will only change his or her behavior when properly motivated either in response to catastrophe or in a series of small steps. We will try to create an environment to precipitate the small steps.

Keeping Sessions Brief

Except in situations posing an immediate threat to life or limb, we suggest that practitioners limit contact with patients who arouse negative emotions to no more than 10 or 15 minutes, regardless of the complexity of the problems or lists of complaints. During that time the practitioner is encouraged to integrate medical and psychosocial concerns, treating the patient in the context of the total life situation. If there are too many problems for one visit, the patient can be brought back the following week. This strategy has the additional advantage of demonstrating the practitioner's interest. It addresses the patient's needs in a supportive manner. Patients will feel less rejected (and these patients are highly skilled at getting clinicians and others to reject them) if they are provided with frequent brief sessions. Ultimately this will result in much better utilization of time, since lengthy and frustrating sessions of miscommunication are avoided. Over time, patients will learn to organize the details of their stories to fit into the time available. Practitioners may have to take charge quite directly by saying something such as "I can hear that you have several things that really bother you. You have some abdominal pains that come and go. You feel all shaky inside and are upset that there is so little cooperation at home. That sounds like a lot for you to deal with. What, specifically, were you hoping *I* would do for you today?"

Approaching the Situation Differently

As we have pointed out previously, reframing problems as opportunities for growth and the development of skills is healthy. So, rather than thinking, "Oh, good grief, Mrs. Brown is on my schedule. I hate to see her since she has numerous problems, doesn't take her medicine, never feels grateful, never gets better or stops complaining," we can think, "Oh, it's Mrs. Brown. I feel sorry that she is so needy. Seeing her will give me an opportunity to practice some of these new techniques I'm learning. I will let her talk for about two minutes. I will paraphrase what she has said so she will know I listened. Then, after I find out what is going on in her life and acknowledge her suffering, I will ask her to concentrate on one specific problem and try to get her to identify one small change that she can make to make herself feel better. If I can make the time with her more productive, I will feel good. I will aim for one small win and limit the time with her to no more than 15 minutes."

When practitioners learn to reframe situations and take satisfaction from dealing with difficult patients in a smooth and efficient manner, the practice of medicine may well become gratifying again. Seeing people relax and become less anxious, hostile, or demanding is a tremendous experience. As we change our approach, unreasonable patients often become more reasonable.

Understanding the Patient's Emotional Context

Patients are sometimes unpleasant, critical, and hostile. For some, this is a personality style. Many times, however, patients are frustrated because they are not feeling or functioning well or because they experience chronic symptoms. They may be unhappy with obstacles that prevent them from getting what they want, with what they think are arbitrary rules set by unreasonable people or with hassles involved in obtaining care. They may also be tired of being dependent on care providers who seem unable to help them. In response, they become hostile. They are so sure that they will not get their needs met that their attitude and behavior ensure achievement of this self-fulfilling prophecy. However, an appropriate empathic intervention can break this pattern. Acknowledging the patient's frustration instead of demanding that it be held in check immediately changes the situation. Let us look at some practical examples.

THE HYPOCHONDRIACAL PATIENT

Perhaps the most difficult patients to deal with, over time, are the hypochondriacal patients, whose preoccupation with real or imagined illness tries the patience of the most dedicated practitioner.[2–4] Barsky and his colleagues found that hypochondriacal patients are dissatisfied with their physicians, that physicians are frustrated by the patients, and that the use of the term "hypochondriasis" impairs "the physician's accuracy in assessing the levels of the patient's anxiety and depression."[5] Hypochondriacs suffer from anxiety and depression particularly because they exaggerate their appraisal of disease risk, jeopardy, and vulnerability.[3] They define good health as a condition of being entirely symptom-free and consider any symptoms, no matter how transitory, as indicative of sickness.[6] These patients focus much of their time and attention on monitoring their physical symptoms and suffer acutely while being unsuccessful in finding anyone to cure them. Hypochondriacs respond best when scheduled for regular visits at predetermined intervals regardless of experiencing symptoms. This is intended to alleviate their considerable anxiety about the status of their health. For starters, every two weeks is often tolerable for both patient and practitioner. Over time the interval between visits can be increased.

Informing these patients that they will receive regular care whether or not they are feeling acutely ill is the first positive step in managing hypochondriasis. Regular sessions preempt the patient's need to develop new symptoms to engage the practitioner. After acknowledging patients' concerns about their current symptoms and emphasizing that it must be awful to never feel well, it is essential to follow the BATHE protocol during every visit.

These patients may become defensive and insist that the stress in their lives is not what is causing their symptoms. This should not become a source for argument. On the contrary, it is important to agree with the patient and express genuine concern that given how badly the patient feels, it must be difficult to cope with everything that is going on. Then it is important to add that stress has a major effect on all illness. Once elicited, psychosocial data should be recorded so that inquiries can be made about outcomes of situations in the patient's life. This communicates that the practitioner is interested in the patient as a person and not just as a collection of disease symptoms. The patient does not have to be sick to get attention or a response. As the relationship progresses, the practitioner may wish to explore the patient's unrealistic expectations regarding his or her state of "health."[6]

As we have said, it is important to acknowledge patients' physical suffering and to allow them a reasonable amount of time to discuss it, to prescribe symptom relief, but always to put things back into the context of the patient's life: "How does that affect your ability to spend time with your grandchildren?" "What can you do to maximize enjoyment during the times when you feel reasonably good?" "What might you do to distract your mind and give you at least some temporary relief from your worry?"

Over time, this approach may offer these patients the opportunity to focus on other aspects of life aside from their physical complaints. Previous life experience may have led these patients to believe that care and attention could only be gotten through illness-related behavior. Now there are alternatives. By structuring visits regularly and including broader aspects of the patient's experience, the practitioner can treat the hypochondriac quite successfully. We again caution practitioners not to let the length of the session exceed their own tolerance for contact with this type of patient. With some patients it may be necessary to limit the time to seven or eight minutes. The session would start with the practitioner making this clear: "Mrs. Brown, we have about eight minutes. Tell me what you are most concerned about this week." Since there are regularly scheduled visits, each session can focus on one or two problems. Our experience has been that patients respond very well to this type of treatment. After a while, they will tolerate longer periods between visits but will usually need to be seen at least once every six weeks, or they will regress. It is also important to allow these patients to keep at least one or two symptoms. Watzlawick[7] has pointed out that it is critical to always allow patients an unresolved remnant.

THE CHRONIC COMPLAINER

There is a subtle difference between hypochondriacs who are truly anxious regarding the state of their health (sometimes referred to as the "worried well") and chronic complainers,[13] troublesome patients who have multiple complaints, feel the need to be seen frequently, and fit into the category of entitled demanders, so aptly described by Groves.[1] These patients rarely improve and never seem to appreciate the efforts that the practitioner makes on their behalf. It would appear obvious that these patients need their disease in order to function at all, as seen by the following example:

> Mary S. has been seeing Dr. L. for almost eight months on a regular basis. She is a 47-year-old, divorced, obese, white female, with moderately well-controlled hypertension, who also complains of insomnia and a variety of aches and pains. Mary had been laid off from her job as a factory worker and been put on temporary disability payments. She is very angry because her benefits are about to expire and she has problems paying her rent, argues constantly with her 21-year-old son who lives with her, and feels that her married daughter and son-in-law treat her badly. Mary talks loudly and fast. It is as though she wants to get 20 minutes of conversation into a 10-minute session. Dr. L. usually feels as though he has been assaulted, or perhaps run over by a lawn mower, after spending any amount of time with her.
>
> Routine lab work and careful examination have convinced Dr. L. that Mary's problems are primarily stress-induced, stress that she generates for herself and others. He has developed a clinical style that allows his patient in the first minutes of the interview to complain about whatever is bothering her most, after which he takes control and examines one problem in detail. After monitoring medications and "laying on hands," in the process of a brief physical examination, Dr. L. wonders what Mary could do differently in a specific interaction with her son. He sees her regularly, every two weeks. Her improvement is obvious, and she is starting to become aware that she has power to make things happen, and not just by being demanding. There are even indications that since she feels accepted she is learning to listen (a little).

The body of contemporary literature focusing on somatization disorders continues to grow.[2,8-16] The basics of psychosomatic medicine were first proposed in a 1943 article by Franz Alexander[17] in which he explained that some patients experiencing internal conflicts but not free to express certain emotions, such as anger, fear, frustration, neediness, or sorrow, developed the physical symptoms that were concomitants of the emotion. Psychiatrists contend that once these emotions can be expressed directly, the need to somatize will decrease.[18] Studies evaluating utilization of outpatient medical services have consistently documented high consumption by patients who somatize and experience their psychological distress as physical.[19-22]

We know that the stress response (including self-induced stress, as it is with the chronic complainer) will activate physiological reactions that are acutely felt and can become chronic and ultimately precipitate organic problems. Patients experience physiological symptoms that result from sympathetic arousal that does not get discharged productively. Many patients do not know how to get any kind of care or attention without complaining. Sadly, when their complaints are not effective, they persevere and complain louder and longer, further increasing their own as well as others' stress.

Life stress has been shown to be predictive of increased medical care utilization for all patients, but particularly for somatizers.[23] The distinction between psychiatric and medical treatment for these patients has become irrelevant.[24,25] However, to be effective, treatment needs to focus on re-education and stress management as a way to help patients manage their symptoms.[26] Until patients become aware of the mechanisms involved and the power to ameliorate their reactions, they are trapped. Anyone who is trapped or pushed into a corner is not very nice to deal with. The effectiveness of cognitive stress management interventions that help people to reinterpret situations, thereby changing the actual emotional reaction, becomes obvious. Therapeutic interventions by practitioners that empower patients and slowly, over time, convince them that they can affect their health, emotions, the course of their lives, and get their needs met directly rather than by complaining about symptoms are extremely effective. When the chronic complainer bemoans the fact that his wife offers him no sympathy, the practitioner can respond, "I can see that that is very difficult for you. What is it, specifically, that you want from your wife?"

Patient: "I want her to pay attention to me."

Practitioner: "That makes sense. Does she pay attention when you tell her about your pain?"

Patient: "No, she ignores me. Then she starts complaining about her headaches."

Practitioner: "I see. Can you think of something you could do to change the situation?"

If the patient responds negatively, it is important not to argue. Power struggles are not useful. When we convince patients that they are wrong, we lose, because we damage the patients' self-esteem. In Chapter 1, we pointed out the enormous power that is attributed to practitioners. This power can be used therapeutically to great advantage. It can also be used detrimentally, to diminish the patient. It is best to try to get the patient to commit to doing one small task that has a positive and realistic potential. When the patient says that his wife complains about her headaches, perhaps the patient could give her the kind of sympathetic response that he desires. It would certainly get her *attention*.

One of the great challenges of outpatient medicine is that practitioners have no control over what patients do after they leave the office. If patients are not committed to the treatment plan, they will sabotage the practitioner's best efforts. Practitioners must convince patients about the importance of changing a behavior, that change is possible, and that there is a payoff for trying. Assignments must be broken down into modest, feasible tasks, and then small wins will accumulate, reinforce the patient's efforts, and make big differences.

BEHAVIORAL TREATMENT FOR ANXIETY

According to the late Gabe Smilkstein MD,[27] "Anxiety is the enemy of health." Anxiety is a signal that the body sends to warn of danger. The signal is real and its manifestations scary, but the danger is often nonexistent or self-induced. Nevertheless, this fear signal results in massive somatic arousal. It is the discomfort with and further fear of arousal that make this a clinical problem. When patients experience somatic arousal they tend to engage in behavioral avoidance of situations that precipitate these sensations. They also assume certain cognitions (catastrophic beliefs) that have been linked to depression and symptom severity in somatizing patients.[28] These behavioral and thought patterns result in worsening the lack of self-efficacy, anticipatory anxiety, and hypervigilance.

There are many effective treatments for anxiety, both pharmacological and behavioral. It is imperative to assure the patient that the varied symptoms are both real and frightening but that they can be managed. Although prescribing medication is always an option, when patients learn to control their symptoms through relaxation techniques, cognitive restructuring, meditation, regular exercise, or desensitizing themselves through predetermined hierarchies of feared situations, their levels of arousal will diminish.[29] Patients can be taught diaphragmatic breathing and progressive muscle relaxation and be asked to practice these techniques for 15 minutes twice daily.

TABLE 7.1 Diaphragmatic Breathing

Instruct patients to start by fully exhaling, pushing their belly button into their spine, and then to breathe in deeply by letting their abdomen expand and engaging their diaphragm. After holding the breath for a few seconds, the process is repeated. Fully exhaling, then inhaling by expanding the abdomen. Also known as "belly breathing," this should be done very slowly and practiced several times a day for about 15 minutes. As they breathe out, let them think about letting tension go. As they breathe in let them think about filling up with calm energy. Mastery of the technique can be achieved in about two weeks. **Once learned, "belly breathing" can be used both as first aid for stress, or when anxiety strikes and to manage chronic stress or anxiety.**

The practitioner can also encourage patients to become aware of their thoughts, to monitor those thoughts for distortions (generalizing, "awfulizing," and "catastrophizing"), and to substitute more positive or functional thoughts. Once the patient becomes aware that the negative and frightening ideas, not the actual situation, are precipitating their anxiety, the practitioner can teach the patient

to challenge these thoughts by reflecting on one or more of the following questions from the work of Beck and Emery.[30]
1. What is the evidence?
2. What is another way to look at the situation?
3. All right, what if that does happen?

This is another area where *bibliotherapy*,[31] such as reading books from Appendix B, can be very helpful. When patients acquire psychological insight into their condition and master techniques that make them feel that they can control their symptoms, they will feel safer. There will be less need to be vigilant against danger. Sometimes it will be necessary for patients to make major life changes to escape from situations that are truly destructive. Having the practitioner to help sort out the options can be very supportive.

For symptomatic relief while the patient is learning skills or preparing to make life changes to reduce the source of the anxiety, Beck and Emery[30] suggest using the A-W-A-R-E technique to label and manage anxiety. The elements of A-W-A-R-E are as follows:

TABLE 7.2 The AWARE Technique

A	–	Accept the anxiety
W	–	Watch your anxiety. Rate the anxiety on a scale from 0 to 10, and watch it change
A	–	Act with the anxiety. Act as if you are not anxious. Breathe deeply and slowly
R	–	Repeat the steps until the anxiety goes down to a comfortable level
E	–	Expect the best.

The "AWARE" protocol can be written on a prescription blank and given to the patient. Having a structure for dealing with the symptoms of somatic arousal puts the patient back in control. Practitioners can also apply the strategy for themselves when dealing with anxiety producing patients.

Stress Management and Cognitive Therapy

We would like to be absolutely clear as to what is involved in the practice of stress management. The first prerequisite for managing stress is to become aware that one is experiencing tension. This can be done by gently scanning areas of the body where tension is usually felt – for example, between the shoulder blades, at the neck, temples, or in the lower back. The overt symptoms that mark acute stress are rapid and shallow breathing, muscle tension, and racing thoughts. Therefore, stress management consists of deliberately taking slow, deep breaths, relaxing the muscles, and modifying the thought process. As mentioned earlier, diaphragmatic breathing and progressive muscle relaxation are easily learned techniques that only require brief daily practice over a period of perhaps two weeks to be mastered (*see* Table 7.1).

Racing thoughts can be managed with cognitive-restructuring strategies. These techniques require patients to pay attention to their perceptions and challenge their interpretations of various situations; in other words, to change their stories. Patients learn to monitor their thought patterns and to become aware of and recognize when their thinking is unduly negative. They can then modify their unrealistic assumptions (horror stories) and substitute more realistic, appropriate, and adaptive versions. The combination of relaxation training and cognitive restructuring is the essence of Cognitive Behavioral Therapy (CBT).

TREATING THE SUBSTANCE-ABUSING PATIENT

Substance abuse continues to be a major problem in society although the "drug of choice" may vary over time.[32,33] Treating the alcohol or narcotics abuser is difficult because, by definition, these patients do not exercise control or take responsibility for their behavior. Four questions useful for making a diagnosis of alcoholism focus on asking patients whether they have ever felt they should *cut down; are annoyed by criticism, have guilt feelings,* and *ever needed an eye-opener.* The acronym "CAGE" helps the practitioner to recall the questions.[34] The questions can be modified to detect problems with other types of chemicals. When screening elicits evidence of a problem, the practitioner may wish to refer the patient to an appropriate treatment program.

If a practitioner wishes to personally manage the treatment of this type of patient, the first step is for the patient to accept responsibility for allowing social drinking to get out of hand or for attempting to run away from, rather than deal with the pain or problems in his or her life. The first constructive step in overcoming a substance abuse problem is for the patient to admit helplessness to control the addiction and to accept help from an outside source.[35] Recognizing that drinking has created an additional problem rather than being a solution for dealing with life's stressors is the first step in the patient's recovery. Substance abusers are not generally capable of mustering the resources to solve problems by themselves. Therefore, the patient must agree to accept help and to diligently follow the instructions of the practitioner. A firm contract must be made with the patient committing to abstinence from the drug of choice (or other non-prescribed chemicals), following the practitioner's orders explicitly, and agreeing to honestly report any infringement of these conditions. Firm limits must be set, and the contract made dependent on strict adherence. The patient's involvement in a 12-step support group is likely to increase the odds of success dramatically.

Helping Patients to Change their Behavior

Whether patients are abusing alcohol or tobacco, maintaining a sedentary lifestyle, eating the wrong foods, or engaging in other destructive health habits, practitioners must be mindful of the fact that people will not change their behavior until they are ready to do so. This means that the individual has to see the necessity or benefit, consider it possible, and feel it is safe to do so (i.e., it will not result in a loss of "face"). Clearly, using power tactics is futile. We recommend two strategies.

First, if a behavior is destructive, the practitioner should inquire at every visit whether the patient has "thought about" changing the particular behavior. If the patient says "yes," this can be reinforced with "Good. That's the first step. You might think about when you might want to actually do it." If the patient says, "I've tried and I can't," the response must be "You just haven't been successful **yet**." Use of the word "yet" may help patients attain the "contemplative stage," which is a prerequisite for changing behavior based on Prochaska and Di Clemente's transtheoretical model of change.[36]

The second strategy, based on motivational interviewing,[37] involves giving patients a homework assignment to construct a decision balance. This means listing all the benefits and risks of the current behavior and the perceived benefits and risks (losses of pleasure, friends, etc.) of the changed behavior. These can then be discussed at the next visit. Until patients recognize that the benefits of changing their behavior clearly outweigh the costs and effort involved, no lasting, positive outcome can be expected.

THE DEPRESSED PATIENT

Having to spend time with depressed patients can be very depressing. It is even more depressing to realize that depression *not* diagnosed or treated by primary care practitioners has always been highly associated with long-lasting symptomatology, decreased quality of life, and suicide.[38] A systematic review of suicide prevention studies found that physician education in depression recognition and treatment and the restriction of access to lethal methods were the only strategies that reliably reduced suicide rates.[39]

So what's involved in recognizing depression? In general, using the BATHE technique will elicit the patient's affect. If there is cause to suspect that the patient may be depressed, there are two questions that may be used to follow-up and screen for depression. The 2 questions are:

1. In the past month, have you often been bothered by feeling down, depressed or hopeless?
2. In the past month, have you often been bothered by having little interest or pleasure in doing things?

A "yes" answer to either or both is a positive screen for depression.[40]

Over 30 years ago, Klein and Seligman[41] demonstrated conclusively that getting people to successfully accomplish small tasks can reverse the learned helplessness (the story based on past experience that there is nothing to be done to escape a bad situation), which is the correlate of depression. Not all depressions are major ones, but even mild to moderate depressions negatively affect people's lives. Recent research documents the association between depression (and anxiety) and the prevalence of obesity.[42] Additionally, adults with depression tend to smoke, binge drink, drink heavily and be physically inactive.[42] Depression can be treated very effectively using brief sessions. Since there is something contagious in the negativity, heaviness, hopelessness, and neediness expressed by these unhappy people, it is important to set realistic expectations for both patient and practitioner. The patient can be expected to suffer but can be encouraged to make some small changes, minute ones if necessary.

Thus, in treating a depressed patient, we first give the patient permission to be depressed. We do *not* suggest that these patients should feel any differently than they do. If they could, they would. We do *not* focus these patients on the positive features of their lives. That only sets up resistance and guilt. We do *not* point out that other people also have horrible problems. Depressed people do not care about the experience of others. We *do* tell the family to stop trying to cheer the patient up. Patients who are depressed and are told to look on the bright side of things, or to count their blessings, often feel misunderstood, wrong, ungrateful, unworthy, or any number of unpleasant feelings, which exacerbates their depression. Instead, we agree that it seems as though *right now* things are really bad and state that we can understand that the patient would feel awful. Sometimes, if we are lucky, the patient will actually respond with something positive. Perversity is an endemic human quality.

Certainly, if necessary, the practitioner can prescribe an antidepressant. However, while waiting for the medication to take effect and subsequently along with the medical treatment, behavioral suggestions and cognitive therapy will be very effective. Psychotherapy and pharmacotherapy have been found to be equally efficacious.[43]

Behavioral treatment might start by suggesting one activity that will give the patient a subjective sense of control:

"I want you to get some exercise, take a brisk walk, perhaps 10 minutes, twice daily. It is not required that you enjoy it, you just have to do it."

"Do one small thing for yourself each day." "Make a list of all the tasks you have to do and feel that you can't. Then do just one, the one that takes the least time." "Forget about mornings, you probably will feel rotten, but plan to do one constructive thing every afternoon."

If there has been a previous history of depressive episodes, it is useful to ask, "What sort of things did you do previously that helped you to feel better?"

Cognitive therapy consists of challenging the negative assumptions and generalities that the patient makes. The practitioner will agree that right now things look very bad but there is no evidence to show that they will always be that way. Focus on the fact that the patient has an illness and that the illness will resolve. Whenever the patient makes a negative statement, the practitioner can edit the statement by inserting the word "yet." "Yes, I understand that you have not been able to motivate yourself to exercise, yet." "No, your appetite has not improved, yet." The implication that things will change – that the patient is not stuck – is very powerful. The practitioner's confidence stirs hope in the patient. Anxiety may be the enemy of health, but *hope is the antidote for depression.*

Depressed patients often believe that the world has to be a certain way before they will be able to function adequately, and they become immobilized in the interim. Cognitive interventions focus on defining the specific problem, devising one or more solutions, and helping patients cope a bit better with whatever is going on in the meantime. A homework assignment might specify that the patient walk at least 30 minutes daily, do something pleasurable no less than once each week, and read the first three chapters of David Burns's *Feeling Good*[44] (*see* Appendix B). The reading assignment can be enhanced at the next visit by having the patient report on what was learned.

Patients who are depressed seem to see the world through very dark colored glasses and focus endlessly on the worst aspects of their situation, thereby making themselves feel worse. This worrying and wallowing is not constructive. Labeling worrying and wallowing for what they are and setting strict limits (perhaps five-minutes every hour – set a timer!) on these activities is an effective intervention. The practitioner must not expect to change the patient's situation but must contract to see the patient regularly, be supportive (lead to the patient's strength), prescribe and monitor medications (if appropriate), and encourage physical exercise.

THE GRIEVING PATIENT

Grief work can usually be accomplished in six to eight sessions. Whenever a patient appears to be overreacting to a current loss, an unresolved grief reaction may be contributing to the severity of the response. The practitioner needs to probe and ascertain if this is true. If so, it is important to explain the necessity for the patient to complete the mourning process and to acknowledge how tough this can sometimes be.

Grief work can be very difficult for the patient. First of all, because it is painful. Moreover, although all people feel some ambivalence toward the significant others in their lives, most people are uncomfortable with the anger that is generated when they experience abandonment by a loved one through death or other circumstances. Conversely, when a troubled relationship ends in divorce or separation, patients may be uncomfortable when they experience a sense of loss and longing for the positive aspects of the liaison. It is important that patients accept these feelings and as they review the significant aspects of the lost relationship.

The six or eight sessions do not necessarily have to occur weekly. In a resistant patient, either because of reluctance to experience the intense pain or because the patient is in denial about the significance of the loss, the practitioner can simply bring up the subject briefly every time the patient is seen for any medical problem. However, ideally, the patient will be cooperative and willing to work. Because grief work does require a thorough airing of the issues and reminiscing about important details, homework in the form of writing about the person or the details of the loss can be very helpful.[45] Talking to relatives or friends, reviewing snapshots, and visiting significant places can be very beneficial. The 15-minute session with the practitioner is then used to highlight important understandings. The patient is doing the work on his or her own time and simply recording the progress with the practitioner. As stated previously, the grieving process involves reviewing the significant aspects of the loss, coming to terms with both the good and bad aspects of what is gone, feeling the pain, accepting the finality of the event, and finally letting go.

Anniversary reactions are extremely common, and patients benefit from being warned to expect a variety of somatic symptoms and mood shifts around the anniversary date of a loss or other significant event.[46] Effective treatments simply involve encouraging patients to feel and accept their pain, rather than trying to shut it off. It is helpful to explain that pain comes in waves, will pass, and does diminish over time. It is important to state explicitly, "You will not always feel this way." In the meantime, all that is required of both the patient and the practitioner is just to be there.

THE SUICIDAL PATIENT: A MEDICAL EMERGENCY

When working with depressed or grieving patients, suicide is always a potential risk, but we will never know if they are suicidal if we do not ask. These patients are experiencing such high levels of emotional pain that the desire to turn off this pain may make the option of killing themselves appear to be quite attractive. Suicide continues to be a leading cause of death worldwide.[47] Research suggests that approximately one-half to two-thirds of individuals who committed suicide visited a physician within 1 month of taking their lives.[48]

In general, serious consideration of suicide corresponds with serious feelings of poor self-esteem, lack of social support, and lack of hope. People who talk about suicide will do it, if their attempts to get help fail. But then, people don't always volunteer their intentions. Consider the following case:

It was a first visit for Dr. Nguyen, who was only in his second year of training in Family Medicine, with a 30-something-year old single, Hispanic-American male who stated he wanted to have some blood tests done since he had not seen a doctor in years. The patient appeared generally healthy, except for some scaly, itchy plaque on his arms and legs that looked like psoriasis. He was a non-smoker, reported that he drank occasionally but not significantly, worked as a salesman and lived with his girlfriend and his 8-month old daughter. Dr. Nguyen noted that the patient seemed anxious but considered that normal since this was his first visit. However, the patient appeared unduly concerned about his health, which was basically normal. Dr. Nguyen decided to BATHE the patient. He inquired: "What is going on in your life?" The patient reported that he felt overwhelmed, had lots of pressure to perform at work, and, also at home to take care of the new baby. He added that he had no time for himself, had no friends, and that the previous night he had felt like hanging himself in the garage. Dr. Nguyen did not ask the patient how he felt about that because he understood that the patient felt overwhelmed, under pressure and socially isolated. At this point, Dr. Nguyen thought, "Man, he's really serious about killing himself!"

Without further prompting, the patient went into a description of a suicide plan, including the intention to write a suicide note to his daughter saying that he loved her and that this was not her fault. He reported that he had not told anyone about his suicidal thoughts or his plan excepting just now, to the doctor. Dr. Nguyen took the patient seriously because of the detailed strategy. He kept the patient calm by listening and reassuring him that it was good that he had decided to come to see the doctor. He also told the patient that he was glad that the patient had not killed himself. The patient responded that he still felt overwhelmed. The physician then proceeded with a physical exam, which was essentially normal. After discussing the case with his preceptor while having a nurse stay in the exam room with the patient, Dr. Nguyen called the suicide hot line. He then informed the patient that he was going to be taken to the ER at the hospital because suicide is considered a medical emergency. The patient appeared confused and asked to call his girlfriend who was shocked. Dr. Nguyen then spoke with the girlfriend on the phone explaining the nature of the medical emergency and that the patient would be given the required help at the hospital.

After being assessed in the Emergency Room the patient was transferred to a local inpatient psychiatric facility for 2 days. He then returned for a follow-up visit with Dr. Nguyen and stated that he was doing well. He appeared well. He related that being hospitalized gave him a couple of days off to assess his situation. He now realized that his family really does care about him and was giving him increased attention. Dr. Nguyen asked him whether he had further thoughts about suicide to which the patient replied that he had no ideation or plan. He was no longer depressed or suicidal.

During a subsequent conference, Dr. Nguyen commented that if he had never asked, he would have never known about the potential suicide. When seeing patients with or without depressive symptoms, primary care physicians do not consistently inquire about suicidality. In a study by Feldman and colleagues suicide was only explored in 36% of 298 encounters with overtly depressed patients in primary care.[49] The use of the BATHE technique detected this patient's suicidal ideation and plan. Thus, BATHE may be a valuable tool for suicide assessment. Dr. Nguyen referred the patient for weekly 30-minute sessions of cognitive behavioral therapy to help him establish a relationship with his infant daughter, manage his anger better and communicate more effectively

138

with his girlfriend. After only two weeks, the therapist reported that the patient responded exceedingly well and was applying the concepts he learned quite consistently and productively.

In this case, a young physician used a routine BATHE inquiry to detect a patient's intention to kill himself. The physician was able to arrange immediate transfer for emergency treatment and then follow through with a referral to a mental health practitioner for collaborative care.

The Practitioner's Support Is Key

As long as the patients have not made a specific plan, primary care practitioners can treat potentially suicidal patients quite effectively. When patients feel that someone is really concerned about them, they will change the story that there is *no one* in the world who cares and that *everyone* would be better off if they were dead. The practitioner acknowledges that suicide is always an option, that it even may seem desirable at a given time, but that once exercised, suicide excludes all other options. Since it is always better to keep one's options open, the practitioner might say, "I hate to see you use a permanent solution for what may turn out to be a temporary problem. Let's keep your options open. Why don't we see how you feel in a few weeks? Let's take it one day at a time, and see if together, we can find a better way to deal with your situation."

It is imperative to double check whether the patient has made a plan. If so, the patient must be willing to *commit* to postponing action or as with the patient above, will have to be hospitalized for his or her safety. Even with a potential plan, the therapeutic connection with the practitioner can be powerful enough to overcome the feelings of hopelessness and demoralization leading to thoughts of suicide.

The practitioner who chooses to treat a potentially suicidal patient must be available for that patient should the patient need to feel connected. If the clinician is going to be away and someone else will be on call, the covering practitioner must be informed about the seriousness of the situation and the support that must be given. It is hoped that family and friends will also be mobilized. As an assignment, the patient is told to ask for support from significant others. In the case cited above, the patient's girlfriend had no idea that he was despondent and felt isolated. It is important to have the patient verify a commitment to call at a particular time or to come in for an appointment in two days or whatever time period is mutually agreeable. The patient must be given clear instructions to call at a specific time when the practitioner will be personally available to talk.

Documentation Is Essential

In general, a patient's promise to call or come in at a specific future time can be safely interpreted as a statement that the patient expects to be around at that time. The patient commits to not harming himself or herself in the interim. A note to that effect must be put into the chart: "Patient promises to call tomorrow to check in. Will be seen on Wednesday for follow-up. Will take no action before further in-person discussion. Patient instructed to go to the emergency room if situation worsens." The patient signs the note as evidence of agreement with the conditions.

TREATING CHILDREN

When we say that every patient should be BATHEd, that includes children. It is often fascinating to compare what a child tells us about what is going on to the story that we get from the adults in the family. Often the discrepancy can be used to make an effective intervention. Asking children what is happening in their lives, how they feel about it, what troubles them the most, and how they are handling it and then giving them empathy establishes wonderful rapport. Sometimes we can help them to interpret their situations differently; other times we can intervene with the parent using the principles outlined in Chapter 6.

Young children or children who are reluctant to talk can be asked to draw a picture. Since children usually draw what is important to them, asking them to tell a story about the picture provides an easy way to get useful information and to connect with the child.[50] Asking a child to draw a person[51] or to draw a family is a lovely way to keep a child occupied while examining a parent and can be used to screen for developmental or situational problems. The practitioner asks the child to "tell me about this family." The practitioner can ask about the various people in the drawing. How do they feel about each other? What makes them happy? What makes them sad? What do they do when they get mad at each other? The practitioner can ask the child, "If you could change one thing, what would it be?" Except in unusual circumstances, interventions focused on changing the parents' behavior toward the child are more efficient and effective than trying to engage the child in a psychotherapeutic relationship. When a case is difficult, referral to a collaborating family therapist is an option to consider.

Treating Adolescents and Young Adults

The practitioner should inform parents of young teenagers that it is important to establish a separate relationship with the adolescent. Every visit must include time without the parent in the examining room. Establishing confidential relationships with teenagers is paramount in gaining their trust and respect. Continuity in the relationship also helps. Teenagers can be BATHEd around issues of home, school, peers, and their ambitions.

Since the potential for violence and abuse in our society is so high, Peter Stringham, a pediatrician working in the Boston area, suggests that in addition to routine questions about illness, friends, religion, smoking, alcohol, drugs, gambling, sexual activity, depression, and suicidal thoughts or actions, it is important to ask, "Have you ever been forced to have sex against your will?" and "How many pushing and shoving fights have you had with anyone in the past year?"[52] Screening for violence in relationships and teaching assertive alternatives are important interventions that primary care practitioners can make.

It is important to support adolescents' self-esteem and to acknowledge the difficulty of sorting out the many choices that have to be made on a daily basis. The practitioner can act as a trusted advisor or encourage the adolescent to find another adult (not the parent) to fulfill that role. Teenagers can also be advised to keep journals to record their feelings and experiences. If teenagers are angry with their parents they must be cautioned not to self-harm through cutting or self-destruct through unduly risky sexual or drug related behavior just to get back at their parents. In general, parents should be told to stop nagging (since it does not do any good) and stop criticizing (since it does harm). Teenagers and young adults respond equally well to our techniques. Practitioners in college health services have reported exceptionally good results using our methods, an example of which follows:

Dr. A. assumed that Ken was fairly healthy because this was his first visit to the office since his college health physical and he was now a member of the junior class. His presenting request that "I would like to have my blood pressure checked" was a bit unusual, particularly when, as a matter of routine, the college nurse had checked his vital signs and found them to be textbook "normal." After dispensing with the usual amenities Dr. A. got to the issue of Ken's concern about his blood pressure and quickly ascertained that his problem was fatigue, which he interpreted as a sign of "low blood pressure." Further questioning about the duration and nature of his fatigue, his work and sleep habits, and related symptomatology was less productive except that Dr. A. got the sense that something was disturbing Ken. He struck gold when he used the BATHE technique:

Dr. A.: "Ken, what is going on in your life?"

Ken: "Well, Doc, my roommate and his girlfriend are using our room to do their thing; it's gotten to the point that I can't even get in there to get a good night's sleep."

Dr. A.: "How do you feel about that?"

Ken: "It makes me really angry; I am paying for that room, and I can't even use it."

Dr. A.: "What troubles you the most about that?"

Ken: "Well, he claims that he is not keeping me out; both he and his girlfriend suggested that my new girlfriend and I join them but we're just not ready to take that step in our relationship."

Dr. A.: "How are you handling that?"

Ken: "Not well, I mean I am not getting very much sleep, and I'm getting more and more irritated. It's beginning to affect my grades as well as my relationship with my girlfriend."

Dr. A.: "That must be very difficult for you."

When Ken acknowledged that it was, Dr. A. suggested that he think about what other options he could exercise. Ken returned the following week to report that he had a long talk with his roommate and that they had come to an agreement that Ken was comfortable with. Ken was feeling very good about himself and how he handled the situation. He thanked Dr. A. for his support. He said that he could not have done it without him.

Just supporting Ken and making him aware that he had other options empowered him to do what he had to do to solve his own problem, which is generally the case. In Chapter 9 we will discuss how to reconcile the needs of the patient with those of other family members.

SUMMARY

In taking care of difficult patients, awareness that these patients are attempting to solve problems in the best way they can is helpful. Setting limits regarding the length of the visit and the number of problems discussed and reframing the situation as an opportunity for learning help the practitioner cope.

Hypochondriacs suffer from anxiety and depression, particularly because they exaggerate their appraisal of disease risk, jeopardy, and vulnerability. Scheduling them for regular appointments and exploring the context of their lives along with their symptoms are effective treatment. Their suffering is acknowledged, and they are allowed to retain one or two symptoms. Chronic complainers are recognized as needing their disease, but they are encouraged to make small changes that help them feel more in control of their lives.

To successfully treat substance abusers, strict limits must be set. Patients will only modify their behavior when they are ready to do so, but strategies can be employed that will encourage them to contemplate making a change. Overt symptoms indicating stress generally involve rapid and shallow breathing, muscle tension, and racing thoughts. Stress management generally consists of deliberately taking slow, deep breaths, relaxing the muscles, and modifying the thought process. Depressed patients must be given permission to be depressed, while being encouraged to make small changes in the circumstances of their lives. Homework assignments can include physical activities as well as reading assignments. Grieving patients are advised to examine the significant aspects of their terminated relationships and actively mourn their losses. In order to heal, they need to feel their pain, rather than trying to shut it off.

Thoughts about committing suicide combined with a plan to do so constitute a medical emergency. Serious consideration of suicide generally corresponds with feelings of poor self-esteem, lack of social support, and lack of hope. If there is no overt plan for action, the practitioner counters these negative feelings by a show of concern and a commitment to help. A contract is made, and the patient promises to call or come in at a specific time. Clear documentation and backup are required.

Children and teenagers can be BATHEd during a regular office visit. Children's drawings help to facilitate communication with the practitioner. Although it is essential to respect teenagers' confidentiality, it is also important to screen for interpersonal violence and high-risk behaviors and to support constructive anger management.

References

1. Groves JE. Taking care of the hateful patient. *N Engl J Med*. 1978; **298**: 883–7.
2. Oyama O, Paltoo C, Greengold J. Somatoform disorders. *Am Fam Physician*. 2007; **76**(9): 1333–8.
3. Creed F, Barsky A. A systematic review of the epidemiology of somatisation disorder and hypochondriasis. *J Psychosom Res*. 2004; **56**(4): 391–408.
4. Barsky AJ, Ahern D, Bailey D, *et al.* Hypochondriacal patients' appraisal of health and physical risks. *Am J Psychiatry*. 2001; **158**: 783–7.
5. Barsky AJ, Wyshak G, Latham KS, *et al.* Hypochondriacal patients, their physicians, and their medical care. *J Gen Intern Med*. 1991; **6**: 413–19.
6. Barsky AJ, Coeytaux RR, Sarnie MK, *et al.* Hypochondriacal patients' beliefs about good health. *Am J Psychiatry*. 1993; **150**: 1085–9.
7. Watzlawick P. *The Language of Change: elements of therapeutic communication*. New York: Basic Books; 1978. p. 73.
8. Rittelmeyer LF. Coping with the chronic complainer. *Am Fam Physician*. 1985; **31**(2): 211–15.
9. Barsky AJ. Patients who amplify bodily sensations. *Ann Intern Med*. 1979; **91**: 63–70.
10. Crofford J. The hypothalamic-pituitary-adrenal stress axis in fibromyalgia and chronic fatigue syndrome. *Rheumatology*. 1998; **57**(Suppl. 2): 67–71.
11. Heim C, Ehlert U, Hanker JP, *et al.* Abuse-related posttraumatic stress disorder and alterations of the hypothalamic-pituitary-adrenal axis in women with chronic pelvic pain. *Psychosom Med*. 1998; **60**: 309–18.
12. Allen LA, Gara MA, Escobar JI, *et al.* Somatization: a debilitating syndrome in primary care. *Psychosomatics*. 2001; **42**(1): 63–7.
13. Miller AR, North CS, Clouse RE, *et al.* The association of irritable bowel syndrome and somatization disorder. *Ann Clin Psychiatry*. 2001; **13**(1): 25–30.
14. Naliboff BD. Towards a nondualistic approach to multisystem illness. *Am J Gastroenterol*. 2007; **102**(12): 2777–80.
15. De Waal MW, Arnold IA, Eekhof JA, *et al.* Follow-up study on health care use of patients with somatoform, anxiety and depressive disorders in primary care. *BMC Fam Pract*. 2008; **9**(1): 5. (Epub ahead of print)
16. Noyes R Jr., Stuart SP, Watson DB. A reconceptualization of the somatoform disorders. *Psychosomatics*. 2008; **49**(1): 14–22.
17. Alexander F. Fundamental concepts of psychosomatic research: psychogenesis, conversion, specificity. *Psychosom Med*. 1943; **5**: 205–10.
18. Fenichel, O. *The Psychoanalytic Theory of Neurosis*. New York: W.W. Norton & Co.; 1945.
19. Escobar JI, Golding JM Hough RL, *et al.* Somatization in the community: relationship of disability and use of services. *Am J Pub Health*. 1987; **77**: 837–40.

20. Fink P, Sorensen L, Engberg M, *et al.* Somatization in primary care: prevalence, health care utilization, and general practitioner recognition. *Psychosomatics.* 1999; **40**(4): 330–8.
21. Hansen MS, Fink P, Frydenberg M, *et al.* Use of health services, mental illness, and self-rated disability and health in medical inpatients. *Psychosom Med.* 2002; **64**(4): 668–75.
22. Barsky AJ, Orav EJ, Bates DW. Distinctive patterns of medical care utilization in patients who somatize. *Medical Care.* 2006; **44**(9): 803–11.
23. Miranda J, Perez-Stable EJ, Munoz RF, *et al.* Somatization, psychiatric disorder, and stress in utilization of ambulatory medical services. *Health Psychol.* 1991; **10**: 46–51.
24. Mayou R, Kirmayer LJ, Simon G, *et al.* Somatoform disorders: time for a new approach in DSM-V. *Am J Psychiatry.* 2005; **162**: 847–55.
25. Strassnig M, Stowell KR, First MB, *et al.* General medical and psychiatric perspectives on somatoform disorders: separated by an uncommon language. *Curr Opin Psychiatry.* 2006; **19**(2): 194–200.
26. Allen LA, Woolfolk RL, Escobar JI, *et al.* Cognitive-behavioral therapy for somatization disorder: a randomized controlled trial. *Arch Intern Med.* 2006; **166**: 1512–18.
27. Smilkstein G. *Caveat: patient centered care.* Theme-Day Presentation. Society of Teachers of Family Medicine 25th Annual Spring Conference, St. Louis, April 25, 1992.
28. Hassett AL, Cone JC, Patella SJ, *et al.* The role of catastrophizing in the pain and depression of women with fibromyalgia syndrome. *Arthritis Rheum.* 2000; **43**: 2493–500.
29. Barlow D.H. *Anxiety and Its Disorders: the nature and treatment of anxiety and panic.* New York: Guilford Press; 1988.
30. Beck AT, Emery G. *Anxiety Disorders and Phobias: a cognitive perspective.* New York: Basic Books; 1985.
31. Wright J, Clum GA, Roodman A, *et al.* A bibliotherapy approach to relapse prevention in individuals with panic attacks. *J Anxiety Disord.* 2000; **14**(5): 483–99.
32. Johnson RA, Gerstein DR. Initiation of use of alcohol, cigarettes, marijuana, cocaine, and other substances in US birth cohorts since 1919. *Am J Pub Health.* 1998; **88**(1): 27–33.
33. White HR, Jarrett N, Valencia EY, *et al.* Stages and sequences of initiation and regular substance use in a longitudinal cohort of black and white male adolescents. *J Stud Alcohol Drugs.* 2007; **68**(2): 173–81.
34. Ewing JA. Detecting alcoholism: the CAGE questionnaire. *JAMA* 1984; **252**(14): 1905–7.
35. Brickman P, Rabinowitz VC, Karuza J, *et al.* Models of helping and coping. *Am Psychol.* 1982, **37**: 368–84.
36. Prochaska JO, Di Clemente CC. Transtheoretical therapy: toward a more integrative model of change. *Psychotherapy: Res Theory & Pract.* 1982; **19**: 276–87.
37. Miller WR, Rollnick S. *Motivational Interviewing: preparing people to change addictive behavior.* New York: Guilford Press; 1991.
38. Murphy JM, Olivier DC, Sobol AM, *et al.* Diagnosis and outcome: depression and anxiety in a general population. *Psychol Med.* 1986; **16**: 117–26.
39. Mann JJ, Apter A, Bertolote J, *et al.* Suicide prevention strategies: a systematic review. *JAMA.* 2005; **294**: 2064–74.

40. United States Preventive Services Task Force. Screening for depression: recommendations and rationale. *Ann Internal Med.* 2002; **136**: 760–4.

41. Klein DC, Seligman MEP. Reversal of performance deficits and perceptual deficits in learned helplessness and depression. *J Abnorm Psychol.* 1976: **85**: 11–26.

42. Strine TW, Mikdad AH, Dube SR, *et al.* The association of depression and anxiety with obesity and unhealthy behaviors among community dwelling US adults. *Gen Hosp Psychiatry.* 2008; **30**(2): 127–37.

43. Wold NJ, Hopko DR. Psychosocial and pharmacological interventions for depressed adults in primary care: a critical review. *Clin Psychol Rev.* 2008; **28**(1): 131–61.

44. Burns D. *Feeling Good: the new mood therapy.* Revised and updated. New York: Avon Books; 1999.

45. Pennebaker JW, Kiecolt-Glaser JK, Glaser R. Disclosure of traumas and immune function: health implications for psychotherapy. *J Consult Clin Psychol.* 1988; **56**: 239–45.

46. Bornstein PE, Clayton PJ. The anniversary reaction. *Dis Nerv Syst.* 1972; **33**: 470–2.

47. Gaynes BN, West SL, Ford CA, *et al.* Screening for suicide risk in adults: a summary of the evidence for the U.S. Preventive Services Task Force. *Ann Intern Med.* 2004; **140**: 822–35.

48. Luoma JB, Martin CE, Pearson JL. Contact with mental health and primary care providers before suicide: a review of the evidence. *Am J Psychiatry.* 2002; **159**: 909–16.

49. Feldman MD, Franks P, Duberstein PR, *et al.* Let's not talk about it: suicide inquiry in primary care. *Ann Fam Med.* 2007; **5**: 412–18.

50. Gardner RA. *Psychotherapeutic Approaches to the Resistant Child.* New York: Jason Aronson; 1975.

51. Mortensen KV. *Form and Content in Children's Human Figure Drawings: development, sex differences, and body experience.* New York: New York University Press; 1991.

52. Stringham P. Domestic violence. *Primary Care: Clinics in Office Practice: Mental Health.* 1999: **26**(2): 373–84.

CHAPTER 8

Accenting the Positive: Putting an Affirmative Spin on the BATHE Technique

Positive psychology, the study of human strengths and virtues, as a field of scientific inquiry, was initiated by Martin Seligman in 1998,[1] with the aim of catalyzing a change in psychology from a preoccupation with repairing the worst things in life to building the best qualities in life. Until that time, psychology had focused primarily on human problems and how to remedy them, just as medicine largely continues to do today. The goal of treatment has been to ameliorate the 'bad' (depression, anxiety, dysfunctional cognitions) and return the person to a state consistent with the absence of 'bad'.

Paul Hershberger's ground breaking article "Prescribing happiness: positive psychology and family medicine"[2] makes a strong case that although promoting mental health is consistent with the philosophy of family medicine, in practice the focus has been primarily on the diagnosis and treatment of psychiatric problems. It is our sincere hope that we can help practitioners to shift that focus in a more positive direction. So, in this chapter we would like to highlight the importance of focusing patients on the positive aspects of their lives, cite some exciting findings from research that support this notion, and introduce the Positive BATHE as a way to start putting this into practice.

POSITIVE AFFECT INFLUENCES HEALTH

Positive affect refers to the regular experience of feelings like enthusiasm, determination and inspiration. There is an extensive literature associating positive affect as a personality trait with physical health and longevity.[3] One of the more interesting longitudinal studies analyzed the emotional words in the autobiographies of 180 nuns, written when they were entering the convent at age 22.[4] Those young nuns who focused on their happy experiences in their

147

writings went on to live on average 6.9 years longer than those whose writings demonstrated unhappiness. Similarly, in the 35-year longitudinal study of male Harvard students by Vaillant and colleages,[5] the students with more positive attitudes documented by personality tests early in life, experienced better health and longevity as they aged. Positive affect has been associated with increased survival time in AIDS patients.[6] Personality traits constituting resilience have been shown to be protective of health even under negative conditions.[7] Recent studies highlight the striking effects of having positive thoughts.[3] They enhance the ability of the immune system to protect the body, help overcome depression, and promote both physical and mental health.[3] Positive affect is believed to release endorphins that have a tonic effect on organs, which may contribute to health by diminishing autonomic and endocrine activity that might otherwise diminish immune function.[3] Studies also show that persons who experience positive affect tend to socialize more, maintain a higher quality of social ties and observe better health practices than persons whose affect is more negative.[3]

The components of psychological well-being, including autonomy, environmental mastery, personal growth, positive relations with others, purpose in life and self-acceptance have all been linked to physical health.[8] The question becomes what, if anything, can be done to promote a sense of well-being in patients in order to influence their health in a beneficial manner.

Positive Thoughts Enhance Well-being

Studies have shown that people can improve their psychological well-being and positively affect their physical health by cultivating positive emotions at critical times to cope with negative emotions triggered by adverse conditions.[9,10] Resilience can be fostered by promoting healthy adaptation strategies built on engaging positive emotions and relationships.[11] As we have discussed earlier, there are bidirectional relationships between thoughts, feelings and behaviors. People can influence their emotions by changing their thoughts and/or behavior. Positive emotions can undo the physiological effects of negative emotions.[12] Based on these finding it would seem that interviews focusing on helping people recall positive events in their lives would be very beneficial in promoting positive affect and lead to a sense of well-being. This is a technique that has been successfully used in organizational development.

Appreciative Inquiry

Several years ago we became interested in improving morale among our faculty and discovered the technique of "Appreciative Inquiry."[13,14] Appreciative inquiry contrasts the notion that every human system has something within it that works right with the traditional problem solving model that aims to fix what's broken. In meetings, using the traditional model, people spend their time focusing on what is not working. Discussing the negative situation often results in poor moral and resignation to a problem-filled environment. When data collection focuses primarily on failure, a lack of empowerment and feelings of inferiority are generated. In general, addressing problems in a group setting creates a culture of problem-centered improvement. People only pay attention after learning that they have failed.

In contrast, the appreciative model looks at what is working well. It focuses on solutions that have been put into place as well as capabilities, assets and possibilities. Appreciative inquiry has a strategy based on four "Ds": discover, dream, design and deliver. Participants are invited to *discover* the best of what is currently happening, through the telling of positive stories, they are encouraged to *dream* by envisioning the organization the best that it might be, and then the group works to *design* a strategy to achieve that state. Finally the group *delivers* by implementing the necessary changes. Where traditional approaches concentrate on defining problems, fixing what's wrong and focusing on decay, a process that generates negative energy in a group, the appreciative process finds existing solutions, amplifies what works and focuses on life-giving forces. The positive energy that is created in a group setting when these techniques are employed is palpable.

FROM THE TRADITIONAL TO THE POSITIVE BATHE

We know that patients appreciate being asked about the circumstances of their lives and having attention paid to their emotional reactions.[15] However, some practitioners feel that patients who are seen frequently for chronic conditions or return for follow-up, do not necessarily benefit from a repeat of the standard BATHE questions. Or perhaps the clinicians are not comfortable repeating the exact questions at each visit. So, in response to this concern, the exciting scientific findings from the new discipline of Positive Psychology and our experience with Appreciate Inquiry, we recognized the need to create a new model of BATHE. The Positive BATHE is recommended as a therapeutic option for regular use, especially with frequent, routine, chronic care, follow-up visits.

TABLE 8.1 The Positive BATHE

B	–	BEST: What's the best thing that's happened to you this week? Or since I saw you?
A	–	ACCOUNT: How do you account for that?
T	–	THANKFULNESS: For what are you most grateful?
H	–	HAPPEN: How can you make things like that happen more frequently?
E	–	EMPATHY OR EMPOWERMENT: That sounds fantastic. I believe that you can do that.

Eliciting the Positive Aspects of a Patient's Life

When using the Positive BATHE rather than asking about what has been happening in general, we specifically focus the patient on recalling some positive event. "What's the *best* thing that's happened to you lately?" Sharing positive information will ordinarily trigger positive emotions. For the "A" rather than asking about "affect" which would be expected to be positive, we follow that with the question, "How do you *account* for that?" This question is designed to help the patient get in touch with the cause of the positive event. Understanding how to set the stage for good things to happen, especially in interpersonal relationships is critical to improving one's experience. The "T" in BATHE is designed to trigger the question, "What are you most *thankful* for?" We will be discussing some of the extensive literature on the effects of gratitude later in this chapter. "H" triggers the question, "*How* can you make things like that *happen* more frequently?" and is designed to empower the patient to take a proactive role in achieving positive experiences. The sequence is concluded with the practitioner enthusiastically emphasizing, "*That's exciting, I'm sure you'll do it.*"

E.M., a 63 year-old widow with diabetes, hypertension, mild depression, and insomnia was seen for a regular follow-up visit and to renew her prescriptions. After listening to her usual litany of complaints, and going over her current medications, Dr. S. inquired about what was the best thing that had happened to her since her last visit. E.M. looked at him with a quizzical look and replied that nothing good ever happens to her. Dr. S. was not to be deterred. He insisted, "O.K. maybe nothing wonderful, but something nice must have happened in the last few days." Suddenly a big smile crossed her face. "Oh yes," she replied, "I got a letter from my granddaughter. She's 8. She wrote me a letter." "How do you account for that?" asked the doctor. "Well, I guess she wanted to be in touch with me. She likes me." The smile was back. Then Dr. S. wanted to know what E.M. was most thankful for. "I really love that little girl. She is so sweet. I'm grateful that she's in my life. I do wish they lived closer, though." Dr. S. then wanted to know how E.M. could make sure that there would be more positive interactions with this grandchild. The patient replied that she would answer the letter, set up regular phone conversations and plan an extended visit. Dr. S. responded by saying he thought that was an excellent plan and that he was glad she had this to look forward to. He also added that he wanted her to exercise regularly. He suggested she walk at least 30 minutes a day, most days, so that when she went for the visit she would be able to actively play with the grandchild. When the patient left the office, she was still smiling.

Recounting Good Things

There is growing empirical evidence that increasing gratitude is associated with increased happiness and decreased depression. In a 6-group, random-assignment, placebo-controlled internet study, Seligman and his associates found that a simple exercise asking people to list three things that went well each day and their causes increased happiness and decreased depressive symptoms over a six-month period.[16] In using the Positive BATHE, practitioners are asking patients about one thing that went well (B: What's the *best* thing to have happened?) and then asking about the cause (A: How to do *account* for that?)

Herschberger[2] suggests that performing the three good things exercise for one week would tend to alter one perspective on one's life. Besides prescribing it for patients, he recommends it for students, graduate trainees and for physician self-care. We certainly concur that paying attention to the good things in life is a prerequisite for being happy. Asking about one occurrence during a clinical interview promotes a positive step in that direction.

Gratitude, a Marker for Health and Well-being

Research shows that dispositional gratitude is associated with positive affect and a sense of well-being.[17] In survey research involving 2616 sets of male and female twins, Kendler and his colleagues found that the trait of thankfulness significantly reduced the prevalence of depression, anxiety and substance abuse.[18] Until recently, there was little data to document the effect of interventions that promote a focus on thankfulness. In an experimental study, subjects who were asked to keep a gratitude journal on a *weekly* basis exercised more regularly, reported fewer physical symptoms, felt better about their lives as a whole, and were more optimistic about the upcoming week compared to those whose journals focused on hassles or neutral life events.[19] Seligman's group found that fulfilling an assigned task to write a gratitude letter reduced subjects' depressive symptoms for a full month.[16] The "T" in the Positive BATHE focuses patients on what they are most thankful for. This can later be enhanced by homework assignments to keep a journal recording thoughts focused on gratitude or writing thank-you letters to someone who has treated them particularly kindly.

Positive Character Traits

Positive character traits and the signal strengths that produce them have been an important area of scientific investigation in Positive Psychology.[16] Character strengths fall under categories of wisdom and knowledge, courage, humanity, justice, temperance and transcendence (finding meaning in life).[1] Each of these has specific traits that contribute to manifesting the strength. For instance, creativity, curiosity, love of learning, open mindedness, and perspective are all particularly salient in acquiring wisdom and knowledge.[1] One of the more interesting findings of Seligman's[16] study, was that participants who identified five of their signal strengths and were then challenged to use one of the signature strengths in a new way, were happier one month after completion of the task than they had been at baseline.[16] When practitioners pose the "H" question, "How can you make things like that *happen* more frequently?" they focus patients on using signal strengths in a new way.

THE POWER OF FORGIVENESS

Forgiveness is one of the characteristics listed under the character trait of temperance.[1] Blaming others for one's misfortunes and sustaining hostility and anger have been shown to be physically and mentally harmful.[17] When subjects in an experimental condition were asked to imagine forgiving a real-life offender they experienced significantly improved cardiovascular (heart rate, blood pressure) and sympathetic nervous system functioning as shown by skin conductance and brow muscle (corrugator) electromyograms than did participants in the non-forgiving conditions.[20] The four physiological reactions measured in this experiment provide a window into what happens to the body when people harbor negative thoughts about an offender and may actually point to mediators between forgiveness and health.[20] Although, people cannot undo past offenses, changing the story about the offense and the offender, and learning to forgive, can allow a change in emotional and physiological reactions leading to improved health implications. This is important information for practitioners to share with patients.

> Ruth S. had had a long-standing feud with her twin sister, dating back into childhood. The sister, Fran, was more outgoing and popular in school and more successful in getting both Mom's and Dad's attention. Ruth never felt that she could measure up. She nurtured her resentment for years. Family gatherings were torture. She became depressed and also abused pain medication. After she discussed her experience with her family physician who was weaning her off her prescription analgesics, Ruth was asked to write about her relationship with her twin. After several weeks of journaling, she was able to work through the emotions related to her childhood. She accepted the hurt and pain that she had experienced and understood that Fran was just being who she was. She decided it was time to forgive her sister. She recognized that the resentment and negative feelings related to the past that she was harboring were hurting her more than they were hurting Fran. In fact, they were destroying her health. Once she decided to let the resentment go, she felt much freer and became more outgoing. Several years later, when their Mom developed dementia and had to move into a nursing home, Ruth and Fran regularly visited her jointly and Ruth looked forward to their weekly time together with pleasure.

Studies have shown that people who continue to feel vengeful or unforgiving after being injured are prone to depressive symptoms.[21] Holding on to grudges is not good for our cardiovascular system either.[20] Coming to forgiveness is an active, deliberate process that can be taught.[22] It can be accomplished by journaling, or writing about the situation as a homework assignment. Coleman[23] outlines a six-step process for achieving forgiveness.

1. Try to specifically identify the hurt (loss of love, self-esteem, control or influence.
2. Confront the one who injured you (actually or using imagery).
3. Come to some understanding of why this came to pass. (Put yourself in the other's shoes.)
4. Engage in a dialog where you take both sides.

5. Make an active decision to forgive. Take a leap of faith.
6. Totally let go of your pain and resentment.[21]

Although no one chooses to be hurt by other people, we know that personal injuries and interpersonal transgressions may ultimately lead to positive effects. Possible benefits include realizing one's inner strengths, renewing one's spirituality, finding new appreciation for one's life, improved interpersonal relationships, increased wisdom and a constructive readjustment of one's priorities. Michael McCullough and his colleagues have shown that writing about the benefits of an interpersonal transgression not only helped people to come to forgiveness, but encouraged cognitive processing that led to more positive thoughts toward those who had injured them.[24] This is an exercise that can easily be replicated.

OTHER POSITIVE COGNITIVE STRATEGIES

When prescribing happiness, Hershberger[2] introduces the concept of "satisficing" meaning achieving an outcome that is "good enough" in contrast to "maximizing" which aims to achieve the best possible outcome. Not everything that we do requires that extensive research be done to learn about all the possible options and then to pick the one that is clearly most advantageous. Once patients figure out what they want, they can be encouraged to find a readily available solution, rather than a perfect one. When expectations are more reasonable, they are more likely to be met. Hershberger[2] points out that when doctors choose not to prescribe the latest and most expensive antibiotic, because a more common generic alternative is "good enough" they are clearly "satisficing."

In general, having realistic expectations will result in a greater likelihood of their being met and the accompanying positive affect. This also relates to the patient/practitioner relationship. Waters and Sierpina[25] have pointed out that in working with pain patients, it is important to have patients figure out what they passionately care about and will work for. By focusing patients on desired positive outcomes, rather than symptoms and problems, patients' autonomy and self-responsibility are enhanced and positive energy is generated. Patients no longer expect the practitioner to "fix" something that may not be "fixable," rather they work together to achieve the goals that the patient has specified.

Seeing Obstacles as Stepping Stones to Success

Learning to change one's behavior and thinking is not a one trial achievement. Therefore, when patients report that things have not turned out as they had hoped, rather than seeing this as a failure, it can be reframed as a learning opportunity. What occurred that was unexpected? What might the patient do differently in this situation the next time? What has worked in the past? In his book *Learned Optimism,* Seligman[26] shows how individuals can also become more optimistic. He suggests that choosing optimism leads to less depression, more achievement and better health. Positive expectations can become self-fulfilling prophecies. However, it is important to recognize realistic limits to what can be achieved within the scope of one's control over events and the resources that are at hand. Still, hope is one of the signal character strengths. Hope is defined as expecting positive things in the future, working to make them happen and believing that a good future is something that can be brought about.[1] This is a prescription to be regularly shared with patients.

SUMMARY

Positive psychology is the scientific study of ordinary human strengths and virtues. This chapter highlights the importance of focusing patients on the positive aspects of their lives, provides evidence-based support and introduces the Positive BATHE. Positive affect, the regular experience of feelings like enthusiasm, determination and inspiration, is associated with physical health and longevity. Positive thoughts enhance the ability of the immune system to protect the body, help overcome depression, and promote both physical and mental health.[3] Persons who experience positive affect tend to observe better health practices than those whose affect is more negative.

Appreciative Inquiry is a technique that focuses participants on what is going well in an organization. They *d*iscover what is working; *d*ream about the best that can be; *d*esign a strategy; and then *d*eliver the positive result. The Positive BATHE is a therapeutic option recommended for use with patients in frequent, routine, chronic care, or follow-up visits. It is designed to focus patients on the positive aspects of their lives. The B stands for BEST: "What's the *best* thing that's happened to you this week?" or ". . . since I saw you?" The A stands for ACCOUNT: "How to you account for that?" T stands for THANKFULNESS: "For what are you most grateful?" H stands for HAPPEN: "How can you make things like that happen more frequently?" and E stands for EMPATHY or EMPOWERMENT: "That sounds fantastic. I believe that you can do that."

An exercise requiring patients to list three good things that have happened each day may lead to a more positive outlook on life. Feelings of gratitude have been associated with improved health status. Patients can be encouraged to identify their signal character strengths and learn to use them in new ways. Forgiveness, letting go of old resentments and grudges, usually results in improved mental and physical health. Patients can be taught a process that leads to achieving forgiveness. They are required to identify the specific hurt, confront the perpetrator in person by imagery, recognize why this happened, create dialog taking both sides, make a decision to forgive, and then completely let go of their pain. When people forgive, their emotional and physical reactions change. Writing about the beneficial effects of a personal injury on one's life can facilitate the process of forgiveness. The concept of "satisficing" is introduced as a strategy for reducing the stress inherent in having to always find the optimal solution to any problem. The difficulty in making permanent changes in one's behavioral and cognitive patterns is acknowledged. However, every negative outcome can be used as a learning experience. Realistic optimism can be expected to lead to positive outcomes and improved quality of health. Hope should be prescribed regularly.

References

1. Peterson C. *A Primer in Positive Psychology.* New York: Oxford University Press; 2006.
2. Hershberger P. Prescribing happiness: positive psychology and family medicine. *Fam Med.* 2005; **37**(9): 30–4.
3. Pressman SD, Cohen S. Does positive affect influence health? *Psychol Bull.* 2005; **131**(6): 925–71.
4. Danner DD, Snowdon DA, Friesen WV. Positive emotions in early life and longevity: findings from the nun study. *J Pers Soc Psychol.* 2001; **80**: 804–13.
5. Peterson C, Seligman MEP, Vaillant GE. Pessimistic explanatory style is a risk factor for physical illness: a 35-year longitudinal study. *J Pers Soc Psychol.* 1988; **55**: 23–7.
6. Moskowitz JT. Positive affect predicts lower risk of AIDS mortality. *Psychosom Med.* 2003; **65**: 620–6.
7. Bonnano GA. Loss, trauma, and human resilience: have we underestimated the human capacity to thrive after extremely aversive events. *Am Psychol.* 2004; **59**: 20–8.
8. Ryff CD, Singer BH. *Emotion, Social Relationships and Health.* New York: Oxford University Press; 2001.
9. Fredrickson BL, Mancuso RA, Branigan C, *et al.* The undoing effect of positive emotions. *Motiv Emot.* 2000; **24**: 237–58.
10. Aspinwall LG, MacNamara A. Taking positive changes seriously. *Cancer.* 2005; **104**(11 Suppl): 2549–56.
11. Masten AS. Ordinary magic: resilience processes in development. *Am Psychol.* 2001; **56**(3): 227–38.
12. Tugade MM, Fredrickson BL. Resilient individuals use positive emotions to bounce back from negative emotional experiences. *J Pers Soc Psychol.* 2004; **86**: 320–33.
13. Fitzgerald S, Murrell K, Miller M. Appreciative Inquiry accentuating the positive. *Business Strategy Review: London Business School.* 2003; **14** (Spring ed.).
14. Swee DE, Stuart MR, Afran J. *Appreciative Inquiry and Wisdom Circles for Transforming Routine Faculty Meetings Into Constructive Group Development Activities.* Seminar, STFM Annual Spring Meeting, Toronto, Canada 2004.
15. Leiblum SL, Schnall E, Seehuus M, *et al.* To BATHE or not to BATHE: patient satisfaction with visits to their family medicine physician. *Fam Med.* 2008; **40**(6): 407–11.
16. Seligman MEP, Steen TA, Park N, *et al.* Positive psychology progress: empirical validation of interventions. *Am Psychol.* 2005; **60**(5): 410–21.
17. Bono G, McCullough ME. Positive responses to benefit and harm: bringing forgiveness and gratitude into cognitive psychotherapy. *J Cognitive Psychother.* 2006; **20**(3): 147–58.
18. Kendler KS, Liu XQ, Gardner CO, *et al.* Dimensions of religiosity and their relationship to lifetime psychiatric and substance use disorders. *Am J Psychiatry.* 2003; **IGO** (3): 496–503.
19. Emmons RA, McCullough ME. Counting blessings versus burdens: experimental studies of gratitude and subjective well-being in daily life. *J Pers Soc Psychol.* 2003; **84**: 377–89.

20. Witvliet CV, Ludwig TE, Vander Laan KL. Granting forgiveness or harboring grudges: implications for emotion, physiology and health. *Psychological Sci.* 2001; **12**(2): 117–23.

21. Brown RP. Measuring individual differences in the tendency to forgive: construct validity and links with depression. *Pers Soc Psychol Bull.* 2003; **29**: 759–71.

22. Worthington EL, Scherer M. Forgiveness as an emotion-focused coping strategy that can reduce health risks and promote health resilience: theory, review, and hypotheses. *Psychol Health.* 2004; **19**: 385–405.

23. Coleman PW. The process of forgiveness in marriage and the family. In: Enright RD, North J (eds.). *Exploring Forgiveness.* Madison, WI: University of Wisconsin Press; 1998. pp. 75–93.

24. McCullough ME, Root LM, Cohen AD. Writing about the benefits of an interpersonal transgression facilitates forgiveness. *J Consult Clin Psychol.* 2006; **74**(5): 887–97.

25. Waters D, Sierpina VS. Goal-directed health care and the chronic pain patient: a new vision of the healing encounter. *Pain Physician.* 2006; **9**(4): 533–9.

26. Seligman MEP. *Learned Optimism: how to change your mind and your life.* New York: Pocket Books; 1998.

CHAPTER 9

Handling Special Situations, Staff, and Assuring Self-Preservation

Having looked at ways to manage some of the most difficult patients, and the importance of focusing attention on the positive incidents in our lives, a myriad of collateral problems remain. Not the least among those problems is dealing with family members, especially when they present a self-righteous or divided front. Are there ways to handle these situations smoothly? We think so. Effective strategies rely on applying the principles discussed earlier. This chapter will also outline constructive approaches that can be taught to nurses, receptionists, and other staff members to help cut down on patients' frustration and anxiety. Finally, we will address the application of psychotherapeutic (cognitive) principles as they apply to the practitioner. Managing our own stress and using every problem as an opportunity for personal growth are prerequisites for successfully coaching patients in these skills.

HANDLING DIFFICULT FAMILY MEMBERS

Dealing with the patient's family can be one of the most rewarding or most frustrating aspects of practicing medicine. Often family members will call and provide unsolicited information about a patient or make suggestions about treatment. The confidentiality issue is clear in this situation. Practitioners may not share information about the patient, but it is perfectly all right to listen to information offered by the family. When factual discrepancies arise, loyalty to the patient and concern for the patient's welfare must guide any response. Sometimes practitioners may feel stressed by the lack of clarity regarding their relationship to family members. In general, however, it is important to avoid power struggles and confrontations. Although family members can be assumed to have their own agendas, the practitioner is not responsible for figuring out their issues or making judgments as to their merit.

157

The Art of Verbal Aikido

When patients' relatives raise concerns about treatment issues, avoiding power struggles and not offending the family are important considerations. We recommend learning the art of "verbal aikido." Aikido is a Japanese martial art, sometimes referred to as "the dance." When a person who is skilled in aikido is attacked, instead of absorbing a frontal blow, the automatic response is to step to the side and turn quickly, join with the attacker, and follow along in the direction of the attack. Then, after a few seconds, the aikido master gently turns both himself or herself and the attacker around, so that they are both going in the opposite direction. After this, the master can gracefully disengage or knock the attacker out.

Verbally, this translates into always acknowledging the legitimacy of others' requests or positions. It catches them off guard and leaves them open to hearing what the practitioner has to say. By first showing respect for the family member's position and anxiety, the practitioner defuses any potential defensiveness. So, when making treatment or discharge plans or discussing anything with a family member, including the behavior of teenagers, we suggest that the practitioner automatically start with the phrase, "I can hear how concerned you are, but . . . (then state your case)." If it is more comfortable, you may prefer to say "I know you care a great deal about your mother (father, husband, son, aunt, niece, grandmother, etc.), but . . .."

It is irrelevant whether you actually subscribe to the above statement. Making the statement is an effective strategy that gets you the other person's attention and positive receptivity. The same thing can be accomplished by starting with the phrase "I agree with you that . . . (and find some part of their suggestion that you can accept)."

Start by Expressing Agreement

People hear better when someone starts by agreeing with them. The critical issue here is that the more difficult and demanding family members are – regardless of whether you see any merit in their suggestions or even feel that they have a legitimate stake in the outcome – there is nothing to be gained by direct antagonism. Starting by agreeing with them puts them into a frame of mind to listen to you. That is what makes this technique so powerful.

You may say to yourself, "That drunken bum hasn't given two hoots about his mother in the last five years. Why should he tell me how to treat her?" You may be absolutely right, but it will be more difficult to deal with the son if you confront him with that. Instead, saying, "I can see how concerned you are. This must be very difficult for you. I am really glad you are letting me know what you would like me to do, but my impression (clinical judgment, good medical practice) demands that I do such and such. I will keep you informed." deprives the other person of ammunition for attacking you. In a later section, "Confronting the Patient," we will discuss the technique for direct confrontation, which should be done only when absolutely necessary. A second verbal aikido technique is to respond to every unacceptable request with the phrase, "I *wish* I could do that!" This implies that you are not arbitrarily saying "no," that the request is not unreasonable, and that you care about the well-being of the person doing the asking. It is a very good way of disarming people and avoiding endless arguments. If a family member does continue to insist, it is only necessary to repeat "I *do wish* I could do that."

Relieving Guilt Is a Therapeutic Intervention

Another important consideration when dealing with families is to recognize that often there are large elements of guilt. When the son from Chicago suddenly calls you and demands that absolutely everything be done for his father, whom he has neglected for years, it is a clear sign that an attempt is being made to resolve guilt. We recommend that practitioners absolve family members of guilt whenever possible. Guilt often stems from projected feelings of resentment. In any case, however, guilt is such an unpleasant emotion that a concomitant hostility is generated toward the person who "makes us" feel guilty. Actually, guilt and hostility are opposite sides of the same coin. It is always therapeutic to say, "I feel confident that you did as much as you could." That is always true. It may not have been enough for the other person, but if the guilty individual could have done more (given his or her story about the relationship), it would have happened. Do not say, "You have no reason to feel guilty." The guilty person is likely to argue. Just say, "I'm sure that you've expressed your love, as best you could. No one can expect more than that."

Enjoying the Challenge

All these interventions are designed to facilitate communications while allowing us to practice according to our best judgment. As in aikido, instead of meeting opponents head-on and absorbing the impact of direct blows, we go to their side first, and join with them in going in their direction, and then when their resistance has diminished, effectively spin them around and head where we want to go. It is fun. Reframing also helps. Instead of thinking, "Why do I have to deal with all these impossible people?" (and it is clear that some people *are* more impossible than others), we think, "Here is an opportunity to practice my new skills and see how I do." To the upset husband we say, "I know you have Jane's interest at heart and that you love her very much, *but* at this time I must do what she wants. In the long run, that will be very beneficial for her, which I know is what you want."

DEALING WITH FAMILY CONFLICT

In dealing with family members who disagree over goals and strategies, it is of critical importance to acknowledge the legitimacy of each person's position and reaction. Remember they all have different stories. It has been said that no two siblings have ever had exactly the same parents. They have all had different experiences of their family and tell themselves different tales. (They have different selective memories). In trying to achieve some sort of consensus, it is important to help them focus on a superordinate goal – the welfare of the patient. If they cannot agree, then perhaps the practitioner's best judgment of the patient's needs has to prevail. If the practitioner has been supportive of the family and the patient, it is likely that they will agree on this. The practitioner takes responsibility because he or she has control of the treatment. Trying to modify family dynamics is an important challenge and requires creative interventions that are beyond the scope of this book.[1]

The Ubiquitous Zap

In the next section we will discuss the necessity of occasionally confronting patients who are exhibiting unacceptable behavior. In order to accomplish this effectively, it may be helpful to clarify the concept of a "zap," the way people react to being confronted with negative information about themselves that they do not wish to acknowledge.[2]

Any time we confront others with something they really do not want to hear from us, it can be considered a *zap*. Zaps by definition are subjective experiences of the receiver, who will react (or rather overreact) in stereotypical fashion. They will respond by counterattacking, creating a diversion or withdrawing. It is important to recognize this as normal, to be prepared for it, and to not react to a counterattack as if it was a *zap*. Retreats or diversions must also be accepted and appropriately acknowledged before returning to the initial problem can be productive. Sometimes it is necessary to go through several rounds before finally being heard. This insight is helpful in all interpersonal situations involving conflict that must be addressed, in confronting others about unacceptable behavior, and particularly in dealing with difficult patients or their families.

Confronting the Patient

There are times when a person's behavior goes beyond acceptable limits or causes a problem, making confrontation necessary. Under these circumstances, it is important to point out to the individual in what way the behavior is a problem (i.e., how it affects the practitioner, the staff, or the practice) and to suggest a specific correction. Sometimes this is enough, and the person will apologize and make the correction. More often, however, the person will become defensive and abusive and will refuse to discuss the issue. People will react as though they had been *zapped*. As discussed above, we can expect one of three potential behaviors in response to a *zap*: counterattack, retreat, or diffusion. The three responses work as follows:

Counterattack: "Really, Doctor, I want you to know that I have not been pleased with the way that you treated my mother. I think I will ask someone else to take over her care."

Retreat: "I'm sorry, Doctor, I don't have time to discuss it now (or ever). I'm late for an appointment."

Diffusion: "You think that I'm hard to deal with. My son has been giving me so much trouble lately. He has no plans for the future. What do you think is wrong with the current generation?"

Any of these reactions is typical for persons being *zapped*: that is, being confronted and having to deal with something they have been trying to avoid. When counterattacked by the "zappee," it is important for the practitioner to guard against feeling counter-zapped but to switch immediately to active listening and verbal aikido and then to repeat the original message. This is not as difficult as it sounds. When a negative reaction is expected, the practitioner can be prepared to handle it smoothly:

Fielding the counterattack: "Yes, I agree that sometimes you have not been pleased with my treatment choices, *but* you must cease bringing alcohol into the hospital."

The retreat: "Mr. Jones, I know you are in a hurry, *but* I want you to get that blood test done today."

The diversion: "Yes, I can see how frustrated you are with your son, *but* I must have your signed consent for this procedure, now."

And the combination of all three: "Mrs. Smith, I understand that you are angry because I sometimes don't call you back within a reasonable time frame and that your boss makes unreasonable demands on you at work and that you have to leave right now because your babysitter is unreliable; *but* I cannot continue to treat your diabetes, if you will not take your medicine as prescribed."

TRAINING THE OFFICE STAFF

The office staff largely creates the environment that the patient experiences when coming to the practitioner for treatment. In fact, when a patient calls to make an appointment or wants to speak to the practitioner on the phone, the staff acts as the ultimate gatekeeper.

It is important that receptionists and nursing personnel become aware of the effects of stress on patients, as outlined in Chapter 2. They can learn a few simple and effective strategies for managing patient interactions. For example, our receptionist complained that some patients are very difficult and demanding on the phone and that *they* should learn to be more cooperative. However, we know that people who are upset are often unreasonable. It is not useful to focus on the fact that they should not be that way; the reality is that they are. The question becomes "What can be done to make the person feel supported enough so that healthier responses can be expected? How can we deal with unreasonable patients without contributing to our own stress?" In training our staff, we have developed and posted a protocol of "Rules for Dealing with the Difficult Patient" as follows.

Rules for Dealing with the Difficult Patient

1. Breathe.
2. Smile.
3. Remember that the patient is the one with the problem.
4. Always acknowledge their suffering.
5. Patients are often frustrated and/or frightened and you represent an obstacle.
6. You are in control of the situation – they are not.
7. People who feel frustrated, frightened or out of control are not nice!
8. Always support the patient.
9. Tell them that you *wish* you could give them what they are asking for.
10. Continue to be nice – be clear – set realistic expectations – set limits.

Fielding Phone Calls

Sometimes when a practitioner has not returned a patient's call, for whatever reason, patients will become frustrated and abusive of the staff. Although we certainly do not condone this type of behavior, it is not useful for the receptionist to get upset and respond angrily to the patient. What is helpful is for the receptionist to make a supportive statement: "It must be difficult to have to stay home and wait for the doctor to call back, when you have so much to do (or you are feeling so bad)." "It must be hard when you are so worried about Nancy's fever to not be able to reach the doctor right away. Time passes so slowly when you're anxious, doesn't it?" This type of understanding response makes the patient feel supported, connected to another human being who acknowledges the reaction to the stress as being reasonable – which it is!

Creating Realistic Expectations

The second major thing that the staff must be encouraged to do is to help the patient set realistic expectations. It is of little value to get the patient off the phone by saying, "Yes, I'll tell the doctor to call you right away" when the doctor is not back from lunch, is solidly booked with patients all afternoon, and has to make hospital rounds after five o'clock, before going to an out-of-town medical society dinner at 7:30 p.m. Instead, it is better to say that the doctor will probably not be available to speak to the patient and ask if there is a specific question that needs to be answered or if it can wait until morning.

It is important to specify when to expect the call back. The implication is that the patient's time is also valuable and that he or she has other things to do besides sitting by the phone and waiting for the practitioner to call back. If it becomes impossible for the practitioner to contact the patient within the agreed time period, someone else should call and inform the patient *when* the practitioner can be expected to be free.

We like to compare the experience of the patient to our own when we are phoning someone whose line is busy and we are put on hold. It is very reassuring to have a live operator (not a recorded announcement) periodically break in and report that the line is still busy. The wait is no less interminable, but we know that we have not been forgotten. We have a sense of being acknowledged and still being connected. We need to ensure that patients do not feel forgotten and disconnected. By adopting these procedures, angry repeat calls from frustrated patients will be minimized.

Patients in the Office

There are also potential problems related to patients in the office. Because of their particular personalities, the staff finds it extremely difficult to deal with certain patients. Although it is clear that these patients' personalities are not going to change, often their behavior can be managed more effectively. Objectively, these patients' problems may not be serious, but subjectively, their problems are disturbing their precarious equilibrium or they would not be coming to the office for help. The staff needs to understand that under stress patients are not at their best behavior. Unhappy patients may become demanding, unreasonable, angry, impatient, and even rude to the staff, although they often behave in a passive or ingratiating manner with the practitioner on whom they feel dependent.

As laid out above, the staff needs to be able to set reasonable limits, always acknowledging patients' rights to feel as they do and acknowledging their suffering, but asserting the need to control their behavior. The receptionist must inform individuals reciting a laundry list of troubles, insults, and concerns that "I understand that it must be very difficult for you." "I can see how upset you are." "I can hear how angry and frustrated you feel, but . . .." Direct acknowledgment of their suffering relieves patients of continued efforts to convince someone of their plight. Once they have successfully communicated that they are miserable, they will be more apt to be able to hear what others want.

The staff also needs to help patients set realistic expectations for the visit. It is better to say that there will be at least a half-hour wait, when the doctor is running behind schedule, than to say nothing, or worse yet, "The doctor will be right with you," when the doctor will not be right with them. When patients feel as though their comfort is a concern for others, it is more likely that they will be able to respond to the concerns of others.

Care for the Caring

It is important to be mindful of the fact that the staff also needs to feel competent and connected. Frequently acknowledging the contribution the staff is making to the supportive environment of the office will reinforce that practice:

"I really appreciate the way you've handled Mrs. Brown. She must be very difficult for you to deal with." "You must really get tired of having to field all these phone calls when I have trouble getting back to these people in a timely fashion. I am impressed with the grace and skill you use." Positive reinforcement by definition increases the probability of the preceding behavior recurring.

RULES FOR PRACTITIONER SURVIVAL

We have done a great deal of preaching in this book regarding the need to take care of patients' psychological as well as physical needs. We are aware that in order for practitioners to follow through on these practices, their own psychological needs must be met. We will now provide a set of rules that the practitioner can apply to enhance personal psychological well-being. These rules were developed out of our teaching experience. Here are the dozen we have found to be most helpful in practice.

RULE 1: Do Not Take Responsibility for Things You Cannot Control

The implication of this rule is that if we did not have control of the circumstances that created a situation, we do not have to take responsibility for the effect the situation has on others. The practical application of this rule is that when people complain about a situation over which *we* have no control, hence for which we are not responsible, we are able to empathize with their frustration, pain, or other discomfort without becoming *defensive*. Knowing it is not of our doing, we can sympathize with patients about the inflexibility of rules made by hospitals, medical regulators or the government without feeling as though we are required to do anything except comfort the patient. It is a situation over which we have no control. Although the patient's anger may be expressed toward us, it does not belong to us. This awareness allows us to gracefully duck and then support the patient. It is also important to remember that we are not responsible for creating the patient's disease. However, we may (or may not) be able to treat it effectively.

The corollary of Rule 1 is that we must take responsibility for what we can control – our own behavior. And in order to control our behavior, we must first be aware of it. It is also useful to acknowledge and recognize our limits.

RULE 2: If You Do Not Take Care of Yourself, You Cannot Take Care of Others

It is critical that practitioners become aware of their limits and tolerance for certain situations. When we find that we are going on "tilt," it is imperative to take time out to center ourselves. Primary care practitioners need to learn stress management techniques, build a support group, set realistic expectations for themselves, and set limits on the demands of others (gently, of course). Becoming overstressed impairs functioning. Once functioning is impaired, the outcome becomes questionable. This leads to Rule 3.

RULE 3: Trouble Is Easier to Prevent Than to Fix

This concept needs little elaboration. Often one or two minutes spent explaining something or considering the consequences of a potential action can avoid extensive problems. Exploring potential outcomes and worst-case scenarios before making a decision can ultimately save time and aggravation. Doing nothing is often better than doing something, especially when all the data are not in. Applying tincture of time when hasty action might precipitate an unstoppable process is an important option to consider.

RULE 4: When You Get Upset, Tune into What Is Going on with You, and Go Through the Three-step Process

1. What am I feeling?
2. What do I want?
3. What can I do about it?

This strategy for getting in touch with and managing feelings and behavior was presented in Chapter 5. It is an important skill for the practitioner to apply personally. Whenever there is a sense of starting to approach "tilt" – feeling a strong sense of being internally pressured and clearly off balance – we recommend tuning in and labeling the experienced emotion. Is it anger, frustration, impatience, sadness, fatigue, or what? That is Step 1.

Step 2 requires getting in touch with what is actually wanted; for example, "I want the patients to stop being so demanding." "I want my receptionist to be better organized." "I want someone to take care of me, for a change." "I want someone to acknowledge that I am trying to do a good job."

Step 3 requires determining what one can do personally to accomplish what is desired. If we are more responsive to patients, they may actually become less demanding. The receptionist may need some support if this is an unusual style for him or her. However, if the disorganization is chronic and irremediable, the receptionist may need to be replaced. As far as getting someone to take care of us or acknowledging our accomplishments is concerned, we may have to learn to ask for what we want – and then to learn to accept it. Sometimes, there is *nothing* that we can do to get what we want. We cannot get it to stop raining on our parade. We cannot change the past or how someone else is feeling or reacting. We cannot stop people from dying. That brings us to Rule 5.

RULE 5: If the Answer to Step 3, Rule 4 Is "nothing," Apply Rule 1

Rule 1, of course, states that we should not take responsibility for things we cannot control. In this case, since there is nothing we can do to get what we want, we need to accept that fact. We do not beat up on ourselves for not being able to affect something over which we have no power. Given this realization and then recycling Rule 4 usually will result in feeling sad and wishing it was a more perfect world. Since we know there is nothing that we can do to make that happen, this usually results in a feeling of acceptance, smug satisfaction with becoming wiser, and an appreciation of ourselves and our ability to sort out feelings. It has been our experience that when we go through this process, there is generally a strong sense of taking control. This felt sense of control results in reestablishing our feeling of competence which is mutually exclusive to feeling overwhelmed. We are fixed! We feel much better. It works for us just as it does for patients.

RULE 6: Ask for Support When You Need It – and Give Others Permission to Feel What They Feel

This simple strategy affirms the importance of accepting both ourselves and others where we are, given our individual maps and stories. We all need support sometimes, and this need does not imply weakness. Although giving people permission to feel what they feel costs nothing, it is highly supportive. There is recognition of the fact that if they could feel differently, they would.

RULE 7: in a Bad Situation You Have Four Options

1. Leave it.
2. Change it.
3. Accept it.
4. Reframe it.

This strategy was discussed at length in Chapter 6. We cannot underscore too strongly the empowering effect of learning to reframe situations. If there is nothing that we can do to change an uncomfortable circumstance, we can learn to give ourselves points for flowing with it, not upsetting ourselves, using the time to think about options for next time, or any other constructive attitude or behavior. Thus we can turn the undesired situation into a successful learning experience. In any case, a way to program small wins must be found. The small win may simply be deciding not to complain since it is futile and may only make others uncomfortable. Finding a constructive way to look at the circumstances (changing the story) so that it results in a positive personal outcome is the essence of reframing.

RULE 8: If You Never Make Mistakes, You Are Not Learning Anything

Beating up on oneself for an honest, unintentional mistake is not useful. Forgiveness is much more constructive. Being human means we cannot be perfect. However, if we do not *own* (or acknowledge) our mistakes, we cannot learn from them. Mistakes resulting from ignorance or fatigue can be reframed by recognizing that they need to be prevented. See Rule 3.

RULE 9: When a Situation Turns Out Badly, Identify the Choice Points and then Decide What You Would Do Differently Next Time

This rule needs little explanation. The aim is to learn something constructive from a bad situation or unfortunate outcome. If there is nothing that you would change, given a chance to replay the situation, then there is no blame, since circumstances obviously did not work out as expected. However, it is usually a good idea to reexamine the original expectations and evaluate their innate reasonableness.

RULE 10: At Any Given Time, You Can Only Make Decisions Based on the Information You Have

This was also discussed in Chapter 5. It is often useful to postpone decisions when the data are not in, to apply tincture of time, and to talk things through with supportive others.

RULE 11: Life Is Not Fair – and Life Is Not a Contest

It is true that life really is not fair. Once we accept this fact, living becomes easier. We do not even have to feel guilty about talents and possessions that we have that less fortunate people lack. Moreover, life is also not a contest. (Many people live as though it were.) It helps to realize that the important things – such as love, wonder, healing, or reaching one's potential – are on a different dimension from a zero-sum game. This is because the more we allow ourselves and others to be open to these experiences, the more resources become available for everyone. People who feel secure do not need to put other people down.

RULE 12: You Have to Start Where the Patient Is

At any given time, people can only be where they are, given their maps and stories. They are reacting to their perceptions and doing the best they can. If they could be any different, they would be – and so would you. This does not mean that people cannot and do not change. People can and do change but only when they are ready to do so and when it is safe! Being safe means being accepted "as is."

MEDICAL MISTAKES AND SELF-FORGIVENESS

Rule 8, above, suggests that making mistakes creates an opportunity for learning. In our experience practitioners have a very hard time accepting that particular rule, often saying that making mistakes is totally unacceptable in medicine. It may be unacceptable but unfortunately it is common. A recent study of the epidemiology of errors and adverse events in ambulatory care settings estimated that 75,000 hospitalizations, 4839 serious permanent injuries and 2587 deaths occur in the United States each year because of preventable adverse events that occur in outpatient settings.[3] In Chapter 8 we discussed the benefits of coming to forgiveness after being injured by another person. Learning to forgive oneself for errors, especially for errors that have negative consequences for other people, is critical if one is to continue to function and have these traumatic events lead to personal growth and improved performance.

The potential for personal growth and learning can be enhanced through reflecting honestly on both the process and outcome of actions that lead to regrettable incidents. Stuart and McGarry[4-6] have presented a number of experiential seminars dealing with self-forgiveness after medical mistakes. Anecdotal evidence in the form of letters and e-mails from physicians years after the workshops, attest to the efficacy of this process. Using a self-reflection work sheet, participants were asked to write about their most disturbing medical error, briefly describing the nature of the mistake. Participants were then asked to list the emotions they felt after they became aware of the mistake and its consequences. Finally, participants were asked to answer the question: "In retrospect, how might this have been prevented?" After small group processing of the material in the self-reflection work sheets, participants learned about the process of coming to forgiveness. Building on the work of Coleman[7] that was presented in Chapter 8, Stuart devised an outline incorporating the additional steps that must be worked through, in order to deal with medical mistakes and come to self-forgiveness. Participants worked in pairs and found the experience to be an extremely valuable introduction to something that would require more time.[5,6] The process is as follows.

How to Give the Gift of Self-forgiveness

1. Describe the mistake you made.
2. "Name the Hurt." Specifically identify the damage you inflicted both on the patient and on yourself. Define the actual **loss** whether physical, emotional, social (relationship), professional (image), or financial.
3. "Claim the Injury." Feel the feelings. Accept and incorporate the pain consciously.
4. Accept the responsibility. In order to forgive ourselves, we must first blame ourselves.
5. Come to some understanding of *why* this came to pass. Put yourself back into the time of the incident. What was your mental/physical state? What resources were you aware of? How much information did you have?
6. Think about what you might do differently if you had the opportunity to relive the situation. Now describe what you have learned. Commit to applying this learning in the future.
7. Make a decision to forgive yourself while remembering the experience with reverence. Gratefully acknowledge the gift given by the person whom you hurt. Vow to honor that gift.
8. Totally let go of your pain and guilt.

This is not a process that can be completed instantly or even in a brief period of time. However, it is our sincere hope that this outline will provide guidance for a constructive journaling process or be a template for talking with a supportive other. It is only when we work through the grief associated with injuring another and come to self-forgiveness that we can go on and become the effective healers that we are capable of being.

SUMMARY

In dealing with family members, power struggles must be avoided and verbal aikido is used to defuse opposition. People hear better when someone starts by agreeing with them. Relieving guilt is a therapeutic intervention. When having to confront patients or families, practitioners are warned to expect counterattacks, retreats, or diversions.

Training the office staff in supportive psychological strategies is effective, as is adopting enlightened expectations for oneself. It is important to be mindful of the fact that the staff also needs to feel competent and connected. Rules for practitioner survival based on our philosophy, and a structure for achieving self-forgiveness when mistakes have occurred, are presented.

References

1. Doherty WJ, Baird A. *Family Therapy and Family Medicine.* New York: Guilford Press; 1983.
2. Palmer JD. Workshop on Improving Conflict Skills. Unpublished paper, 1977.
3. Woods DM, Thomas EJ, Holl JL, *et al.* Ambulatory care adverse events and preventable adverse events leading to a hospital admission. *Qual Saf Health Care.* 2007; **16**(2): 127–31.
4. Stuart MR. *Self-Forgiveness: Growing from our Medical Mistakes.* Seminar, Forum for Behavioral Science, Chicago, IL. September, 2002.
5. Stuart MR, McGarry BJ. *Growing from our Medical Mistakes: initiating the process of self-forgiveness.* Seminar, 36th Annual STFM Conference, Atlanta, GA. September 21, 2003.
6. Stuart MR, McGarry BJ. *Medical Mistakes and Self-Forgiveness Revisited: how to do it – how to teach it.* Seminar, 37th Annual STFM Spring Conference, Toronto, ON. May 15, 2004.
7. Coleman PW. The process of forgiveness in marriage and the family. In: Enright RD, North J, (eds.) *Exploring Forgiveness.* Madison, WI: University of Wisconsin Press; 1998. pp. 75–93.

CHAPTER 10

Wrapping Up – Integrating Treatments, Modifying Lifestyles, Getting Results

Incorporating therapeutic talk into day-to-day primary care practice can enhance the experience of practitioners, patients, patients' families, and perhaps even society as a whole. Throughout this book we have endeavored to apply scientific principles to highlight the interrelationships among behavioral, emotional, cognitive, social and biological components that impact people's health. As we pointed out in Chapter 1, practitioners have great powers to influence patients' beliefs and behavior. Motivating patients to make constructive lifestyle changes may ultimately be more beneficial than treating disease. For example, the current global rise in the prevalence of obesity certainly presents a serious challenge.[1] In this final chapter, we will first discuss some specific behavioral therapies for common conditions and then focus on the potential effects of applying our techniques to a variety of stake holders.

DEPRESSION AND ANXIETY: CAUSAL FACTORS IN OBESITY

Depression and anxiety have been linked to the prevalence of smoking, obesity and physical inactivity.[2] Men and women with mild, moderate, moderately severe and severe depression are generally more apt to smoke and be physically inactive than those with no depression. In fact, a dose-response relationship exists between depression severity and smoking, obesity and physical inactivity. Primary care practitioners see a lot of patients who are anxious and/or depressed. Primary care practitioners also see a lot of patients who are obese. This suggests the need for a multidimensional and integrative approach to medical care.[2]

PSYCHOSOCIAL VS. PHARMACOLOGICAL INTERVENTIONS

Practitioners always have the option to prescribe medication for problems presented by patients. However, we hope this book will encourage you to use therapeutic talk in addition to or as a substitute for pharmacological treatment, especially for conditions related to lifestyle. Researchers are beginning to explore the efficacy of psychosocial and pharmacological treatments for depression in primary care.[3] After reviewing available data from numerous academic clinical trials, Wolf and Hopko conclude that psychosocial treatments may represent an important alternative to pharmacological treatment, particularly given relatively similar treatment response rates and increased patient satisfaction when these interventions are received.[3] A meta-analytic comparison of pharmacotherapy and psychotherapy treatment in later-life depression also did not show differences in treatment outcome.[4] A Canadian study found that depression could be successfully treated in primary care particularly when the patient was engaged as an active participant in dealing with his or her disorder rather than someone who just complies with treatment.[5] However, the value of listening to patients and recognizing the importance to designing incremental goals that patients can achieve is paramount in the treatment of depression.[6]

Physical Activity and Meditation: Effective Treatment Modalities

Prescribing exercise and motivating patients to follow through with it becomes an important treatment modality. Regular exercise is associated with lower levels of anxiety and depression in all age cohorts,[7] as well as having many other health benefits. Although habitual physical activity has not been shown to prevent the onset of depression, there is significant evidence that increased aerobic exercise or strength training reduces depressive symptoms.[8] Acute anxiety symptoms and panic disorder have also been shown to improve in response to regular exercise.[8] These beneficial effects equal the response to meditation and relaxation. Successful treatments for a wide range of mental and physical health problems are based on the therapeutic action of mindfulness.[9]

Combining Mindfulness and CBT

Mindfulness-based cognitive therapy (MBCT) combines mindfulness training[10] with elements of cognitive–behavioral therapy. Patients are taught to recognize and disengage from states of mind characterized by negative and ruminative thinking and to access and use a new state of mind characterized by acceptance and "being."

Jon Kabat-Zinn[10] is credited with developing mindfulness meditation as a tool for stress management. Meditation, which is simply the practice of uncritically attempting to focus your attention on one thing at a time, has a long history and can take any number of forms.[11] After establishing a posture that is characterized by relaxed attention, and centering oneself by focusing on the breath, meditation can take the form of counting breath going in and out. One can focus by repeating a mantra (a word, or combination of syllables that are repeated) or by gazing softly at an object. When attention wanders it is gently brought back to the object. One can do a walking meditation, focusing on the sensations that are experienced as the feet meet the ground and the muscles in the calves relax and contract. Eating meditation is an excellent way to slow the process and shift one's awareness to the myriad of pleasurable sensations that arise as we contemplate food, place it in our mouths, taste, chew and swallow before digesting. Patients are given an assignment to practice meditating for about 15 minutes twice a day using whatever modality suits them best.

Combining mindfulness with CBT seems to enhance the effectiveness of both techniques.[12] MBCT has been shown to be effective for generalized anxiety disorder.[13] Teasdale and colleagues have repeatedly demonstrated the effectiveness of MBCT for reducing relapse after treatment for depression.[14]

EFFECTS ON THE PRACTITIONER

Adopting an attitude of mindfulness and thinking about the more positive aspects of daily practice should also greatly improve the experience of today's medical practitioner. We hope that when prescribing some of these techniques for their patients, practitioners will choose to incorporate them into their own lives.

Controlling What Can Be Controlled

Trying to practice good medicine within the limits set by government regulations or third party payers certainly can make practitioners feel a lack of control of their circumstances, as well as reducing their confidence in their ability to responsively manage patients' needs. Many reimbursement systems create financial incentives for doing expensive procedures rather than keeping people well and preventing or limiting serious illness. We would encourage practitioners to find ways to reframe these problems as a challenge and growth opportunity. We also recommend increasing their physical activity and decreasing the amount of calories consumed, since these are factors that can be controlled.

Although there is much in life that cannot be controlled, gradually increasing physical activity and decreasing the amount of calories consumed can be accomplished by most people, if it is seen as important. Feeling that one has control over important aspects of one's life has been shown to be an important factor in maintaining and promoting health.[15]

As we pointed out in Chapter 8, a growing body of evidence suggests that enhancing positive attitudes is associated with improved physical health, mental health, and longevity.[16-18] Resilience is cited as a quality that leads to positive adaptation.[19] Realistic optimism, the tendency to maintain a positive outlook within situational constraints, increases the likelihood of desirable and personally meaningful outcomes.[20] Let us look at how this can be applied to the practitioner's own situation.

Responding to a Changed Paradigm

In retrospect, it seems that life used to be simpler. Buckminster Fuller's work has cast out all doubt that "It is fortunate that the Good Lord created the universe exactly divided into the traditional academic disciplines."[21] Just as biochemistry has bridged the gap between biology and chemistry, biophysics has bridged the gap between biology and physics and has much to teach us about immunology. The power of imagery to affect physiological processes is demonstrated daily through biofeedback. We know that how we think determines how we feel and that positive thoughts contribute to positive outcomes. We also know that how we think affects our physical reactions and that feeling powerful or helpless determines our ability or inability to mobilize an effective immune response. The most dangerous state, for our bodies, as well as for our minds, exists when we feel overwhelmed and demoralized.[22,23] The need to adapt to the rapid changes and information overload prevalent in the current practice of medicine, can precipitate a high level of stress. And how do people respond to overwhelming stress? Under extreme circumstances the following happens:

1. they intensify their usual psychological and social coping devices
2. when these devices fail, they experience anger that must be suppressed (or even repressed) or else the sources of existing support will dry up more
3. next, they turn on themselves, blame themselves for not managing better, internalize their aggressive impulses, and develop feelings of guilt and depression
4. finally, they stop trying to cope; instead, they feel helpless and develop a variety of symptoms.

When people give up and stop trying to cope, the prescription is to provide support, making them feel competent and connected by gratifying dependency needs without undermining self-respect.

The strategies described in *The Fifteen Minute Hour* are designed to provide support for practitioners and patients alike. Our "cookbook" approach providing step-by-step instructions for applying effective techniques can lead to improved patient care, and also to enhanced satisfaction, increased income, and personal growth for the practitioner.

Applying a Therapeutic Strategy

For starters, the practicing professional can consider the following questions: How do you feel about what is going on in the medical care delivery system today? Or, how do you feel about how you are practicing medicine today? What do you want? In other words, how do you want to practice? And finally, what can you do about it? Translation: what changes do you have to make in order to be able to do this?

We recommend that you be very clear about the answers to these questions. If there is a desire to practice medicine as it was done in the last century, unfortunately there is nothing that can be done about that. The road goes on. But if the desire is to keep up, be productive, and be successful, to learn and grow, many strategies in this book will contribute to that goal, but only if put into practice.

Achieving Professional Success

As mentioned above, although there are few financial incentives for keeping people well and preventing or limiting serious illness, we feel that there is a moral obligation to practice patient centered preventive medicine. Ideally this should not be a financial drain on the practitioner. By monitoring stressful events in patients' lives on an ongoing basis, problems can be caught earlier and less complicated stages. Practitioners can experience great satisfaction when building a practice based on continuity of care, paying attention to lifestyle and other health-enhancing practices, and providing anticipatory guidance. The most important payoff for the practitioner, however, may ultimately be the joy of participating meaningfully and contributing positively to the quality of patients' lives.

Personal Growth

The final payoff for practitioners adopting and using our therapeutic interventions on a day-to-day basis will be their own personal growth. By applying the principles outlined in this book to their own life situations, practitioners will feel empowered. It will become somewhat easier to juggle professional commitments, family obligations, and personal needs. Practitioners will develop their own sense of coherence and incorporate a rational, flexible, and far-sighted coping style.[24] In order to develop a coherent sense of identity, practitioners need to reflect on their feelings about their careers, relationships with both patients and colleagues, personal relationships, financial and security issues, relationships to the wider community, and ultimately the meaning of life.[25] Becoming aware of the feelings related to these issues, acknowledging wants, and deciding what strategies are available to meet reasonable expectations will lead to positive personal growth. As human beings, we may be organisms affected by our biology and demands from the environment, but we are also agents (subjects who act with intentionality), as well as spiritual beings with our place in the universe.

Moving Toward Self-actualization

When needs for physical survival, security, acceptance, and achievement have been met, practitioners invariably approach that part of A.H. Maslow's hierarchy of needs identified as self- actualization.[26] Maslow pointed out that self-actualized people make full use of their talents, capabilities, and potentialities and develop to the full stature that they are capable of attaining.

Self-actualization results in a more efficient perception of reality and more comfortable relations with it. Self-actualized people do not need to cling to positive illusions, nor do they need to cling to the familiar. They accept themselves, other people, and nature. They are relatively comfortable with the vague and indefinite, and the quest for truth assumes priority over the need for safety.[26] Self-actualized people develop an increased ability to be spontaneous and a code of ethics that is autonomous. Self-actualized people, like good practitioners, are more problem-centered than ego-centered. They exhibit a certain quality of objective detachment and have a need for privacy. They rely on their own interpretation of situations. In other words, they have an internal locus of control.

Other desirable qualities that Maslow[26] cites as characteristic of achieving self-actualization include a continued fresh appreciation of the richness of experience, profound interpersonal relationships, development of a democratic character structure, a sense that means are ends, enhanced creativity, and a friendly sense of humor. People are not born self-actualized. It is a state that is fostered by transcending difficulties and applying the type of therapeutic modalities we are advocating in this book. Adopting these techniques and teaching them to their patients will inevitably have a positive effect on practitioners as well as patients.

EFFECTS ON THE PATIENT

Having discussed from a broad viewpoint the potential benefits likely to accrue for the practitioner who incorporates therapeutic talk into the usual patient visit, let us now look at the potential cumulative effects on patients.

Supporting Health Rather Than Curing Disease

When dealing with patients' problems as outlined in this book, we do not suggest that the practitioner is curing in the traditional sense. It may well be that there is no such thing as a specific disease in the traditional sense or a specific cure. We are proposing that the patient's sense of well-being will be enhanced through the therapeutic interaction with the practitioner. This in turn will support the patient's own healing powers and allow the patient's immune system to function at a normal level of effectiveness.[27] Moreover, from a social perspective, when the patient feels empowered, the patient will behave in ways that will result in more productive interactions with other people.

We are not claiming that we have solutions to chronic problems that have eluded other well-meaning health professionals. Our approach is simply designed to maximize positive outcomes using easily learned, proven behavioral techniques that can be incorporated into the structure of a typical primary care visit and will capitalize on people's strengths.

For the final example to be presented in this book, let us look at the case of Emily M., the type of patient who is characterized by a really thick chart:

Emily M. is a 43-year-old female, with limited education, who came into the office two years previously complaining of chest pain. She brought prescriptions for 13 different medications prescribed by six different doctors. She had been hospitalized numerous times for extensive work-ups of multiple aches and pains for which she had gone to the emergency room and been admitted. Cardiologists, pulmonologists, gastroenterologists, orthopedists, otolaryngologists, and gynecologists had each run their battery of tests from computed tomography (CT) scans and colonoscopy to coronary catheterization, but no one was able to identify the origin of her symptoms. Each consultant added another drug to her regimen and referred her to the next specialist, until she had seen them all. Having run out of sub-specialists, she came to the Family Practice Center.

History revealed that the onset of her various acute pains would correspond with arguments with her abusive, alcoholic, unemployed (disabled) husband. Overall, she presented with the affect and vegetative signs of depression. Dr. S.'s clinical impression was that Emily was suffering primarily from depressive and somatization disorders. He weaned her off all her medications except sublingual nitroglycerin, taught her relaxation techniques, and started her on an activating selective serotonin reuptake inhibitor (SSRI).

Emily was seen once per week for several months, during which time the emphasis was shifted away from her physical pains, to focus on her shattered living situation and family problems. She was encouraged to walk at a moderate pace for 30 minutes at least five days a week. A social worker and a women's self-help group were also involved in her case. Emily was given strict instructions to call the center when she experienced acute pain rather than going to the emergency room. During her regular office visits, Dr. S. attended to her physical complaints without lingering on them and then spent most of the 15-minute session listening to the precipitating factors and new stresses in her life. He offered support and acknowledged her suffering. Using the BATHE technique, he focused her on one problem during each session and wondered what Emily could do to improve matters. Intervals between visits were gradually increased until they were every four weeks. At this time, Emily showed up in the emergency room complaining of chest pain! No acute problem was found.

After that incident, regular visits were scheduled at intervals ranging from every two to every four weeks and Emily improved slowly but steadily. In contrast to the multiple admissions in each of the previous five years, she has remained out of the hospital for two years, except for one hospitalization for hypotonic bowel with partial obstruction at the time of her sister's death. Emily continues to be seen at regular intervals, and although her living situation is no better, she is functioning at a somewhat higher level than before.

In every case, our goals involve helping patients to achieve whatever potential is reasonable for them, *at this time*. For Emily to stay out of the hospital for two years is an enormous accomplishment. Although functioning marginally by society's standards, her current level of adaptation is nonetheless remarkable.

Patients' Realization of their Own Potential

Rather than engaging patients in a relationship that fosters dependency, our support encourages them to maximize their own potential. We focus on their strengths and promote patients' awareness that they are exercising choices at all times, by pointing out that there are always options. It is the patients' responsibility to determine what these options are. Based on the information they have, we encourage them to make the best possible choice at any given time. The implication is that the practitioner and the patient are on the same side, that of the patient. It is through this partnership with the practitioner that patients achieve the confidence to act positively in their own interest.

Enhancing Health

It is generally accepted today that the patient's health is largely determined by what the patient does, that is, the type of lifestyle that the patient adopts, rather than what happens during a visit to a practitioner's office. It is not our intention to quarrel with this statement but rather to encourage the use of strategies and techniques to affect the patient's behavior or lifestyle in positive ways. When a patient is "somatizing" and the practitioner inquires about what is going on in the patient's life, some skeptics may still contend that an uninitiated patient may object to this change of focus. The following example presents one possible response:

> Patient: "You're saying it's all in my mind?"
>
> Practitioner: "No, not at all. What I think is that your body is telling you that you are under stress and really hurting."

We want patients to start listening to their bodies, to monitor themselves and become aware of the precursors to "tilt." In this way they can ease the pressure on themselves without having to become sick.

In recent years, increasing numbers of patients request that their physicians take an active interest in their health and disease processes.[28] Shared decision making and utilization of the practitioner's support can lead to positive health consequences. Patients' sense of well-being will be enhanced, resulting in increased resistance to stressors of all kinds. They may be less susceptible to infections of various sorts, less accident-prone, and able to handle life's problems in more constructive ways. They will become more aware of the impact of their own reactions on others and on the things that happen to them. This type of constructive adaptation can be expected to lead to better physical and mental health.[24] As suggested in Chapter 8, it is also beneficial to focus patients on the aspects of their lives that are going well, by using the Positive BATHE. Finally, it is important to remember that nutrition and exercise have a tremendous impact on people's health and overall sense of well-being.

Reducing the Incidence of Complications

The secondary prevention implicit in our model of practice is quite obvious. Since illness itself generally upsets the balance of psychosocial well-being for patients and their families, the benefits of preventing illness complications are clear. Patients are encouraged to engage their most constructive coping mechanisms, to recognize that they must lower their expectations, to feel supported, and to get their needs met on an ongoing basis rather than forcing the practitioner to manage a series of catastrophes. The trust generated by being cared for and cared about will enhance patients' sense of basic trust in the world (the sense of coherence), which can then be expected to result in improved health consequences.[18]

EFFECTS ON THE FAMILY

It is obvious from the above that improved patient functioning can be expected to positively affect other family members.

Improved Relationships

When patients apply the personal strategies that we have outlined, their relationships within their families, their work settings, and the community in general will improve. People who feel personally powerful both resist being exploited, and also have less need to exploit others. Communication patterns that are open and direct allow problems to be handled in productive ways. This may sound utopian, but we have seen the powerful effects of small wins in mobilizing patients. It is also amazing to see how support enables people to function in their healthy rather than their neurotic modes. When people engage their healthy maps of the world, their altered behavior and positive expectations for their relationships become self-fulfilling prophecies.

Countering Resistance

Of course, specific family dynamics, old conflicts, and competing and seemingly mutually exclusive opinions, agendas, and desires will complicate the effect of patients' newly acquired assertiveness. It is important to counsel patients that they may experience mixed reactions to changes they attempt to instigate. Although family interventions are beyond the scope of this book, we recognize that the patient is a member of a (family) system. Since every part of any system reciprocally affects every other part of the system, when the patient changes certain self-defeating behaviors, this will have significant effects on other family members. After some initial resistance, which may be quite painful, a new accommodation will be made, hopefully with healthier functioning for all.

Potential Benefits of Improved Communications

By encouraging patients to communicate more clearly and directly, they and other members of their family will have less need to manipulate each other by becoming sick or engaging in various other destructive behaviors. As patients apply the practical child management techniques that we have advocated, their children can be expected to grow up with a well-formed sense of security, self-respect, and self-esteem. These children will be comfortable solving problems and making choices. When faced with peer pressure to take on risks, they will automatically consider the worst-case scenario and find ways to maintain friendships as well as their values. A benevolent circle, the essence of primary prevention, will be engaged. People who have an enhanced sense of health and well-being can be expected to treat other people with consideration and respect. Their stories about themselves, the world, and the other people in it will be positive. This can be expected to result in positive interactions with others. If a majority of people were to adopt this view, our society as a whole would benefit greatly.

PUTTING HEALTH PROMOTION AND DISEASE PREVENTION INTO PRACTICE

As part of health maintenance functions, there is a clear directive for the primary care practitioner to screen for depression, anxiety, and stress-related problems and also to help patients manage their reactions to the events in their lives in the most constructive way possible. We have tried to outline how this can be done effectively and efficiently. At a minimum each patient can be BATHEd and given permission to feel whatever feelings are being experienced. Limited information can be provided regarding people's normal reactions to stress and loss. Specific suggestions are designed to help patients manage stress or other troubling situations effectively. Anticipatory guidance to minimize stress inherent in adjusting to expected transitions should become part of routine treatment, while the ongoing relationship with the primary care practitioner provides basic support. Practitioners must learn to ask questions that focus patients on their own strengths. Patients should be encouraged to identify and focus on the positive aspects of their lives.

Appendix A provides 12 effective questions and three excellent responses with which to start to accomplish these goals. The minimal investment in time used in employing these techniques will pay off with maximal therapeutic results. The process will also help practitioners transcend some of the frustrations inherent in the present health care delivery climate, connect meaningfully with their patients, and gain renewed personal and professional satisfaction.

SUMMING IT ALL UP

The last area we'd like to address relates to the laws of ecology. In 1972, Bertram Murray, a Rutgers Professor, wrote an article in the NY Times Sunday Magazine section outlining what ecologists could teach economists. In our opinion this piece is particularly relevant for primary care providers in the 21st Century. These are the seven laws.[29]

1. Everything is connected to everything else.
2. There is no such thing as a free lunch.
3. Nature knows best.
4. Everything must go somewhere.
5. Continuous growth leads to disasters.
6. Competing species cannot coexist indefinitely.
7. The law of the retarding lead.

Let us examine these issues one at a time and see whether they prove helpful.

Everything Is Connected to Everything Else

Information, disease, knowledge, and just about everything else is disseminated through an interconnected series of networks. We exist in relationship to others. Our brains communicate with every cell in our bodies. How we think determines how we feel. Lifestyle choices determine our levels of health and fitness. If the front office is not functioning smoothly, our ability to see patients in a timely manner is compromised. The way we interact with our patients has a direct impact on their healing capacity.

There Is No Such Thing as a Free Lunch

When the drug companies buy, they expect you to listen to their spiel. When doctors prescribe too many antibiotics, resistant organisms develop. Eat more calories than you burn up by activity and you will gain weight. As we use up resources of the planet, and pollution grows, lunch gets more expensive. Our climate is changing. The choices we make on a daily basis have long lasting consequences. Drugs have side effects.

Nature Knows Best

Human beings do not really know all that needs to be known to manage an ecosystem. Doctors do not always know why one person responds to treatment and another does not. Evidence-based medicine deals with statistical probabilities – numbers needed to treat tell us how many people will be exposed to medication to achieve a benefit for a smaller number. They say that every 10 years half of what was taught in medical school changes – only we don't know which half. Good nutrition, exercise, mindfulness, forgiveness, thankfulness, and laughter in good measure, these are the natural healers that will never go out of style.

181

Everything Must Go Somewhere

The waste absorbing capacity of the natural environment is already taxed. We cannot continue to throw things away forever. In health, when we block feelings, keeping them out of our awareness, not just failing to express them, the physical effect can be devastating. Any blockage – of energy, feelings, blood flow or even elimination – think of kidneys shutting down – can be drastic over time.

Continuous Growth Leads to Disasters

More and more money and bigger and bigger practices do not necessarily lead to professional satisfaction. Personal interactions may get lost in the process. Money can become an addiction like everything else. Cancer cells, those that grow without limits, ultimately kill the organism. Too much of anything – food is a good example, does not lead to happiness, just obesity.

Competing Species Cannot Coexist Indefinitely

Economists feel that competition is beneficial because it maintains diversity and allows for choice. In nature, when competing in the same habitat, one of the contending species will ultimately be eliminated from the ecosystem. Whereas those species that cooperate and collaborate, building synergistic communities, survive. Collaborative care is a model whose time has come.

The Law of the Retarding Lead

Adaptive changes and creative solutions do not come from species that are dominant in their niche, but from species and individuals that are forced to be more resourceful because they exist on the fringe. Primary care practitioners are often seen as on the fringe. However, by practicing integrated biopsychosocial patient centered medicine, keeping people as healthy and productive as they can be, primary care practitioners can help to build a medical care delivery system that is truly responsive to societies' needs.

SUMMARY

The global prevalence of obesity and its link to anxiety and depression underscores the need to motivate patients to make constructive lifestyle modifications. Psychosocial treatments can enhance or substitute for pharmacological therapy. Adding mindfulness practices to cognitive behavioral techniques enhances the beneficial effects of these treatment modalities. Practitioners are encouraged to find positive ways to reframe the challenges that today's medical care systems present. Supporting patients and encouraging them to express their feelings will enhance their powers to heal. It may also foster more positive relationships in the greater community. These beneficial effects are also likely to impact families. Regularly BATHEing patients integrates psychosocial and biological systems and becomes an essential part of health promotion and disease prevention. Finally, we present seven laws of ecology that have significance for guiding intelligent medical care.

References

1. Caballero B. The global epidemic of obesity: an overview. *Epidemiol Rev.* 2007; **29**: 1–5.
2. Strine T, Mokdad AH, Dube SR, *et al.* The association of depression and anxiety with obesity and unhealthy behaviors among community dwelling US adults. *Gen Hosp Psychiatry.* 2008; **30**(2): 127–37.
3. Wolf NJ, Hopko DR. Psychosocial and pharmacological interventions for depressed adults in primary care: a critical review. *Clin Psychol Rev.* 2008; **28**(1): 131–61.
4. Pinquart M, Duberstein PR, Lyness JM. Treatments for later-life depressive conditions: a meta-analytic comparison of pharmacotherapy and psychotherapy. *Am J Psychiatry.* 2006; **163**: 1493–501.
5. Bilsker D, Goldner EM, Jones W. Health services patterns indicate potential benefit of supported self-management for depression in primary care. *Can J Psychiatry.* 2007; **52**(2): 86–95.
6. Johnston O, Kumar S, Kendall K, *et al.* Qualitative study of depression management in primary care: GP and patient goals, and the value of listening. *Br J Gen Pract.* 2007; **57**(544): 872–9.
7. De Moor MH, Beem AL, Stubbe JH. Regular exercise, anxiety, depression and personality: a population-based study. *Prev Med.* 2006; **42**(4): 273–9.
8. Paluska SA, Schwenk TL. Physical activity and mental health: current concepts. *Sports Med.* 2000; **29**(3): 167–80.
9. Melbourne Academic Mindfulness Interest Group. Mindfulness-based psychotherapies: a review of conceptual foundations, empirical evidence and practical considerations. *Aust N Z J Psychiatry.* 2006; **40**(4): 285–94.
10. Kabat-Zinn J. *Full catastrophe living: the program of the Stress Reduction Clinic at the University of Massachusetts Medical Center.* New York: Delta; 1990.
11. Davis M, Eshelman ER, McKay N. *The Relaxation and Stress Reduction Workbook.* 4th ed. Oakland, CA: New Harbinger Publications; 1995. pp. 39–54.
12. Coelho H, Canter PH, Ernst E. Mindfulness-based cognitive therapy: evaluating current evidence and informing future research. *J Consult Clin Psychol.* 2007; **75**(6): 1000–5.
13. Evans S, Ferrando S, Findler M, *et al.* Mindfulness-based cognitive therapy for generalized anxiety disorder. *J Anxiety Disord.* 2008; **22**(4): 716–21.
14. Ma SH, Teasdale JD. Mindfulness-based cognitive therapy for depression: replication and exploration of differential relapse prevention effects. *J Consult Clin Psychol.* 2004; **72**(1): 31–40.
15. Schaubroeck J, Jones JR, Jia LX. Individual differences in utilizing control to cope with job demands: effects on susceptibility to infectious disease. *J Appl Psychol.* 2001; **86**(2): 265–78.
16. Fredrickson BL, Levenson RW. Positive emotions speed recovery from the cardiovascular sequelae of negative emotions. *Cogn Emot.* 1998; **12**: 191–220.
17. Maruta T, Colligan RC, Malinchoc M, *et al.* Optimists vs. pessimists: survival rate among medical patients over a 30-year period. *Mayo Clinic Proceedings.* 2000; **75**: 140–3.
18. Danner D, Snowdon DA, Friesen WV. Positive emotions in early life and longevity: findings from the Nun Study. *J Pers Soc Psychol.* 2001; **80**(5): 804–13.

19. Masten AS. Ordinary magic: resilience processes in development. *Am Psychol.* 2001: **56**(3): 227–38.
20. Schneider SL. In search of realistic optimism: meaning, knowledge and warm fuzziness. *Am Psychol.* 2001; **56**(3): 250–63.
21. Fuller RB. *Synergistics.* New York: MacMillan Publishing Co.; 1975.
22. Irwin MR. Human psychoneuroimmunology: 20 years of discovery. *Brain Behav Immunol.* 2008; **22**(2): 129–39.
23. Ader R, Kelley KW. A global view of twenty years of brain, behavior, and immunity. *Brain Behav Immunol.* 2007; **21**(1): 20–2.
24. Antonovsky A. *Health, Stress, and Coping.* San Francisco: Jossey-Bass; 1979.
25. Schmiedeck RA. The sense of identity and the role of continuity and confluence. *Psychiatry.* 1979; **43**: 157–64.
26. Maslow AH. Self-actualizing people: a study of psychological health. *Personality.* 1950; *Symposium.* **1**: 11–34.
27. Glaser R, Rabin B, Chesney M, *et al.* Stress-induced immunomodulation: implications for infectious diseases? *JAMA.* 1999; **281**: 2268–70.
28. McGregor S. Patient roles, power and subjective choice. *Pt Educ & Couns.* 2006; Jan; **60**(1): 5–9.
29. Murray BG. Continuous growth or no growth? What the ecologists can teach the economists. *NY Times Sunday Magazine*; Dec 10, 1972: 38.

APPENDIX A

Twelve Good Questions and Three Good Answers for All Seasons

QUESTIONS THAT HAVE THERAPEUTIC VALUE
1. How do you feel about that?
2. What troubles you the most?
3. How are you handling that?
4. What are you feeling right now?
5. What do you want?
6. What can *you* do about that?
7. What are your options?
8. What is the best thing that can happen?
9. What is the worst thing that can happen?
10. How will that affect your life?
11. What does that mean to you?
12. What, specifically, were you hoping I would do?

RESPONSES THAT HAVE THERAPEUTIC VALUE
1. That must be very difficult for you.
2. I can understand *that** you would feel that way.
3. Under the circumstances, I am sure that you (he, she, they) did the best you (he, she, they) could!

---

* Not to be confused with "I understand how you feel" or "I know how you feel," which are not recommended since they may lead to arguments. No one can accurately know how another is feeling.

APPENDIX B

Recommended Books for Patients

FOR ANXIETY AND DEPRESSION

Burns D. *Feeling Good: the new mood therapy.* **New York: Avon Books; 1999.**
This is Cognitive Therapy in a self-help format. Assign this book, a few chapters at a time, to all your depressed patients. It takes a sensible and effective approach to managing the symptoms of depression. There are inventories, exercises, and clear explanations. With your encouragement patients will benefit enormously.

Jeffers S. *Feel the Fear and Do It Anyway.* **New York: Ballentine Books; 2006.**
This is an absolutely delightful, practical manual to help patients overcome the fears that limit their lives. An easy-to-read and easy-to-apply volume, it contains many exercises that can lead to insights. Patients can choose to work on certain sections and report their progress to the practitioner. Reading this book is wonderful therapy for anxiety of all kinds.

McKay M, Davis M, Fanning P. *Thoughts and Feelings: taking control of your moods and your life.* **Oakland, CA: New Harbinger Publications; 2007.**
This is a workbook of cognitive-behavioral techniques effective for worry control, coping with panic, and overcoming phobias. Patients can also learn to relax, stop unwanted thoughts, change habits, and adjust limited thinking patterns. This latest updated edition includes a chapter on mindfulness. An extremely user-friendly volume.

Young JE, Klosko J, Beck AT. *Reinventing Your Life: the breakthrough program to end negative behavior . . . and feel great again.* **New York: Plume; 1994.**
This book presents evidence-based cognitive techniques for helping patients make major changes in their approach to handling problems. It can facilitate long-lasting improvements from self-defeating patterns of behavior.

Seligman MEP. *Learned Optimism: how to change your mind and your life.* **New York: Pocket Books; 1998.**
This is the definitive volume on Positive Psychology by the author who invented it. Very readable and convincing, this book will help patients develop more positive attitudes and reap enormous benefits.

STRESS MANAGEMENT
Davis M, Eshelman ER, McKay M. *The Relaxation & Stress Reduction Workbook.* 6th ed. **Oakland, CA: New Harbinger Publications; 2008**
This is a complete guide to relaxation techniques that includes chapters on breathing, meditation, visualization, stopping stressful thoughts, time management, nutrition, and physical exercise. This latest edition also includes sections on anger management and mindfulness. This is a particularly effective self-help manual, especially if used with a clinician's supervision. New Harbinger Publications has a whole catalog of self-help materials focusing on every imaginable topic from communication skills (*Messages*), assertiveness (*Assertiveness Training*) and eating disorders (*The Deadly Diet*) to lifetime weight control (*The Body Image Workbook*). Complete listings can be found at: www.newharbinger.com

www.apahelpcenter.org
This useful free website provides the results of the American Psychological Association's survey on the effects of stress on health, as well as articles and tips for dealing with stress.

PARENTING GUIDANCE
Faber A, Mazlish E. *How to Talk So Kids Will Listen, How to Listen So Kids Will Talk.* **20th ed. New York: Avon Books; 1999.**
This little paperback is based on the work of Chaim Ginott MD, and is filled with cartoons and practical suggestions. It will make parents feel as though they have a wise and loving advisor always at hand to help them to deal with normal developmental issues in good-humored ways.

Gordon T. *P. E. T.: Parent Effectiveness Training.* **New York: Crown Publishers Group; 2000.**
This classic still dispenses very good advice. It helps parents to set limits and makes them feel competent in their role.

Satir V. *The New Peoplemaking.* **Palo Alto, CA: Science and Behavior Books; 1988.**
Virginia Satir's philosophical approach is designed to maximize self-esteem in all members of the family. A lovely book to read and enjoy, it nonetheless casts light on the dynamics of healthy and dysfunctional families. It should be available in all public libraries.

FOR DEALING WITH LOSS

Kusher HS. *When Bad Things Happen to Good People.* **New York: Anchor Books; 2004.**

This is a wonderful book to recommend for people who are dealing with tragedy. It is a comforting book that can help patients make sense out of their suffering.

Jewett CL. *Helping Children Cope With Separation and Loss.* Revised ed. **Boston: The Harvard Common Press; 1994.**

This book gives simple techniques for adults to use to help children who experience losses. It includes good background material on stages of grief and effects on children, as well as practical advice from how to tell children that something dreadful has happened, through the shock and denial, to the anger and depression that can be expected to follow. It also gives excellent suggestions for dealing with difficult situations brought on by death, separation, divorce, hospitalizations, major moves, or other traumatic events for children.

FOR EVERYONE

Blanchard K, Johnson S. *The One Minute Manager.* **New York: HarperCollins Business; 2000.**

This book is not just for managers. It helps focus people on what is essential: goals, praise, and complaints. These need to be concisely formulated and communicated clearly. This little book can help patients feel competent and connect with others in positive ways.

Index